Liz Pearson R.D. **and Mairlyn Smith** H.Ec.

the
Ultimate
HEALTHY
EATING
Plan

that still leaves room for chocolate

whitecap

This book is dedicated to my husband Rick, who likes to remind me of the "everything in moderation" rule, my daughter Chelsea, who still wishes fruit roll-ups were part of the four food groups, and my daughter Shannon, who loves broccoli (really!).

LIZ PEARSON
visit Liz's website at www.lizpearson.com

To my grandmother, Euphemia Blundell, who ate grapefruit and oatmeal, drank tea, and lived one month short of her 98th birthday. She taught me that love was in your kitchen.

MAIRLYN SMITH

Edited by JENNIFER GLOSSOP AND LESLEY CAMERON
Proofread by KATHY EVANS
Cover design by ROBERTA BATCHELOR
Interior design by STACEY NOYES / LUZFORM DESIGN
Front cover photographs by FIRSTLIGHT.CA
Back cover photograph by PIERRE GAUTREAU PHOTOGRAPHY

National Library of Canada Cataloguing in
    Publication Data

Pearson, Liz, 1962-
The ultimate healthy eating plan--that still leaves room for chocolate

 Includes bibliographical references and index.
 ISBN 1-55285-334-9

 1. Nutrition. 2. Cookery. I. Smith, Mairlyn. II. Title.
TX355.P418 2002   613.2   C2002-910193-X

The publisher acknowledges the support of the Canada Council for the Arts and the Cultural Services Branch of the Government of British Columbia for our publishing program. We acknowledge the financial support of the Government of Canada through the Book Publishing Industry Development Program for our publishing activities.

Printed and bound in Canada

Contents

Out-of-this-World Delicious Recipes

Appendix

Bibliography

Index

About the Authors

Acknowledgements

Thanks to the Whitecap team who believed in this book and allowed us to make it our own. Thanks to Jennifer Glossop for her meticulous editing. Thanks to dietitians Elizabeth Snell and Lise Smedmor for their insightful review of the manuscript.

Thanks to the many researchers who reviewed specific chapters and provided invaluable input. They include: Eric Rimm (Harvard School of Public Health), Joan Sabate (Loma Linda University), Joanne Slavin (University of Minnesota), Penny Kris-Etherton (University of Minnesota), Jonathan Hodgson (University of Western Australia), Melanie Polk (American Institute for Cancer Research), Sheila Bingham (University of Cambridge), James Anderson (University of Kentucky), Berdine Martin (Purdue University) and Hasan Mukhtar (Case Western Reserve University).

Thanks to my dad for inspiring me to find a career I love and go for it. Thanks to my mom for her incredible assistance with my children. Thanks to my sister Jenny for her never-ending support, encouragement and advice.

Thanks to Mairlyn, my co-author and, even more exciting, my new friend. Mairlyn is a pleasure to work with, has a passion for what she does, and wants this book to succeed as much as I do!

Liz Pearson

March 1998 I first meet Liz Pearson outside The Cookbook Store on Yonge Street in Toronto. We are on our respective book tours and are going to be doing a photo shoot for the *Toronto Star*, featuring our new books. We're both early, and spend about 20 minutes outside the store waiting for Alison Fryer, the store's manager and femme extraordinaire, to arrive. Liz is seven months pregnant, we chat about our books, her upcoming baby, and life in general. I like her, she's friendly, enthusiastic, and gung-ho on her book, *When in doubt eat broccoli, (but leave some room for chocolate)*. The photo shoot goes well and we are in the paper.

July 2000 I'm in Ottawa, sitting in the waiting room of a noon-hour news show, and in walks Liz! We are both working for different food companies and are scheduled to be on the same show! After we get over the shock of bumping into each other in Ottawa we chat about our books and the conversation finally comes around to, "Are you writing another one?" It turns out that we both want to write a book on preventing disease through diet! How weird is that? She looks at me and I look at her, and she says, "I'll call you." If I had a nickel for every time somebody said that to me, I'd be living in Paris right now, drinking red wine and reading a novel in some wonderful little café.

August 2000 There are seven messages on my phone, and one of them is from Liz. I return her call, and two months later we are writing *The Ultimate Healthy Eating Plan (that still leaves room for chocolate!)*

July 2001 One year later! Our manuscript is due in three more days. I have never worked so hard on a project in my life. I'm very pleased with all my recipes, and, bonus, I've lowered my cholesterol. Liz and I talk on the phone 7–21 times a day! Yesterday I didn't call her for three hours and when I did she told me she was in Mairlyn withdrawal!

I am so proud of what we've accomplished. We have both worked our butts off to bring you an exciting new book that can make you feel better and help change your health. When you write a book you put the rest of your life on hold. Here is my thank-you list to the people in my life who helped out while I was holed up in my kitchen: First and foremost my co-author Liz. She's wonderfully supportive and a great person to work with. My son, Andrew, who tasted everything in this book. My partner, Scott, who ate everything in this book! My friends Cathy, Jann, Joanne and Michale, who were there for me, helped me cook, washed dishes, ate stuff and phoned to see if I was okay! And last but by no means least, my assistant Dawn Bone, without whom this manuscript would have been delivered in cryptic writing on the back of recyled scripts to my wonderful publisher, Whitecap, sometime in the year 2004!

Mairlyn Smith

INTRODUCTION

If you were to design the ultimate eating plan, what would it look like? Would it be easy to follow? Would it be based on the most up-to-date scientific research? Would it include super nutritious, disease-fighting foods that could significantly reduce your risk of heart disease, cancer, diabetes, osteoporosis and more? Would the plan be individualized to suit your busy lifestyle and your own individual goals for weight loss or weight maintenance? Would it include out-of-this-world delicious recipes that are also quick and easy to make? Lastly, and perhaps most important, would your plan leave room for chocolate? If you answered yes to any or all of the above, this truly is the ultimate plan for you.

Ultimate Health

You've read that certain foods are good for your health—foods like flax, soy, broccoli, nuts and whole grains. Yet how do you fit all these foods into your everyday diet? How much or how little of these foods do you have to eat to significantly reduce your risk of disease? Does it matter if you eat them cooked, raw, chopped or peeled? The Ultimate Healthy Eating Plan reviews the most current research on foods and their incredible ability to ward off disease. The plan tells you exactly how much of each food to eat each day or each week and gives you endless tips and recipe ideas on how to make it happen. It tells you which fats are actually critical to good health and which fats you should make every effort to eat less of. It ranks various foods in terms of their overall nutrient contribution as well as their ability to prevent disease. The plan uncovers many nutrition myths and misconceptions and includes an update on nutritional supplements. Are certain supplements necessary to prevent disease? And what about beverages? Is green tea better than black? Does a glass of red wine deserve a place in your daily diet? Some of the answers may surprise you. Most important, the ultimate plan is geared to excite and motivate you to enjoy the healthiest diet you can.

Ultimate Ease and Flexibility

It simply doesn't get any easier or better than this. The Ultimate Healthy Eating Plan was designed with your individual needs as top priority. Are you an eating-on-the-run kind of person? Do you sometimes feel that packing a lunch or putting dinner on the table is a major accomplishment? Do you eat more meals at restaurants than at home? What about your weight? Do you need to lose a few pounds or maybe more than a few pounds?

The Ultimate Healthy Eating Plan is simple, easy and designed to suit your lifestyle. In the Putting It All Together section, you'll find a variety of meal plans to choose from. For example, the Summertime Meal Plan uses all the wonderful vegetables and fruit that are available at that time of year. It's geared for hot days when you may want to fire up the barbecue or simply not cook at all. The Wintertime Meal Plan is designed around a more limited selection of fresh produce and also includes lots of great, hot meals for cold, wintry nights. The Weight-Loss Plan clocks in at only 1600 calories per day and yet still contains all the incredible foods and nutrients required for fighting disease and being your best. We think it's the healthiest, tastiest and most practical weight-loss plan ever developed! Lastly, there's the Eating-on-the-Run Meal Plan geared for life in the fast lane. It recommends selections for everything from fast-food restaurants to upscale dining to frozen dinners you pop in the oven. Who could ask for more? It's the ultimate plan for your life and your needs.

Ultimate Taste

The recipes in this book are exceptional. They're not just packed with super nutritious ingredients. They also taste great. The Unbelievably Delicious Raspberry Salad Dressing is, quite simply, unbelievably delicious. The Super Quick Blender Shakes are truly super quick, super tasty and loaded with good nutrition. The Chicken with Mango and Apricots is easy to prepare, yet impressive enough to be served to a king. And the Super Nutritious Chocolate Chip Bran Muffins, made with whole

QUOTE OF THE DAY

"With prolonged life expectancy and the increasing number of elderly, it is predicted that osteoporotic fractures will reach epidemic proportions."

Jasminka Ilich, *Journal of the American College of Nutrition,* December 2000

RESEARCH HIGHLIGHT

Diabetes is a serious disease. People with diabetes are two to four times more likely to die of heart disease. Diabetes can cause blindness, kidney disease and nerve damage. Research suggests that over 90% of Type II diabetes could be prevented if people maintained a healthy weight, exercised regularly, ate a healthy diet and didn't smoke.

grains, flax, prunes and buttermilk, are a guaranteed hit for more reason than one! Mairlyn tested, retested, tested again and fine-tuned each of the recipes in this book until every one of them was sure to get "two thumbs up"—way up!

There are kid-friendly recipes. There are easy, yet impressive, recipes for entertaining (your friends will like them so much, they'll want to jump on the healthy eating bandwagon). There are even recipes you can make in five minutes flat. Best of all, with just a few exceptions, all the recipe ingredients can be found at your local supermarket. It's the ultimate great-tasting eating plan.

Leaving Room for Chocolate

In a recent survey, people were asked what words they would use to describe chocolate—not surprisingly, people used terms such as "awesome, calming, delectable, heavenly, intoxicating, irresistible, sexy and sinful." Few would argue that chocolate is a food loved by many. That's why chocolate is an integral part of the plan (including the weight-loss plan!). You get to enjoy a bit of chocolate almost every day. Options include everything from chocolate chip muffins to chocolate shakes to chocolate pudding. You get to enjoy mini-treats like chocolate-covered raisins and M&M's Chocolate Candies. It was George Bernard Shaw who said, "There is no love sincerer than the love of food."

That's why the Ultimate Healthy Eating Plan leaves room for chocolate and the pleasure it brings.

P.S. Recent research also shows that certain types of chocolate may have potential health benefits (find out more in the Leaving Room for Chocolate chapter).

Body in Motion

The Ultimate Healthy Eating Plan wouldn't be complete without a section on active living—an essential ingredient for optimal health. What's your greatest physical activity challenge? Finding the time to be active? Getting started? Sticking with it? Do you question whether you are doing the right type or amount of exercise? This plan has three goals in mind when it comes to working out—maximal enjoyment, maximal benefit and minimal time. It's the ultimate plan for making active living a regular part of your life.

The Plan

The Ultimate Healthy Eating Plan is super nutritious and fights disease. It's realistic, achievable and the recipes couldn't taste better (especially the ones with chocolate). It's the best investment you can make in you! Here's to happy reading, happy tasting and to being the healthiest you that you can be!

Have fun on your journey,
Liz Pearson and Mairlyn Smith

P.S.
Before starting any new eating plan or exercise program, be sure to check with your family doctor.

HEALTHY-FOR-YOU **FATS**

THE OBJECTIVES OF THE ULTIMATE HEALTHY EATING PLAN ARE TO REDUCE YOUR RISK OF DISEASE BY

optimizing

canola oil | extra virgin olive oil

moderating

soft nonhydrogenated margarine | salad
dressings | mayonnaise | other spreads

FAT IS GOOD!

If you're like most people, you're probably concerned about the amount of fat in your diet. Chances are you feel bad when you eat foods higher in fat and believe you deserve a major pat on the back when you make lower fat choices. While making lower fat choices overall is important for managing your waistline, for disease prevention it's the type of fat you eat that really makes the difference. The research in this area is exciting. By choosing "healthy-for-you fats," you can reduce your risk of heart disease, cancer, diabetes, arthritis and more. The news about fats has never been so good! By the way, if you find fats among the most confusing of all nutrition topics, you're not alone. This chapter will help you make sense of a subject that's frequently difficult to make sense of.

Put Canola On Your List

The Ultimate Healthy Eating Plan recommends canola oil. Here's why:

Alpha-Linolenic Acid Fights Disease

Canola oil is a rich source of alpha-linolenic acid, a type of omega-3 fat. Other excellent sources of omega-3 fats are flaxseed, walnuts and, of course, fish (these foods are all included in the plan and discussed in subsequent chapters). In the Lyon Heart Study, a high intake of alpha-linolenic acid (much of which came from a canola-enriched margarine) was a major factor associated with a 70% reduction in fatal heart attacks. In the Seven Countries Study, those countries found to have the longest life expectancy in the world (Japan and the Greek island of Crete) also reported the highest intakes of this fat.

How does alpha-linolenic acid work? While researchers are still trying to unravel all the remarkable benefits of this omega-3 fat, it appears that:

CLEAR THE CONFUSION
There are three major types of fats in the foods we eat: saturated, polyunsaturated and monounsaturated. Most foods contain all three in varying amounts. There are two main types of polyunsaturated fats: omega-3 and omega-6 fats. For optimal health, most people need to focus more on foods higher in monounsaturated fats and omega-3 fats.

QUESTION OF THE DAY
"Can heart disease be reversed?" Some studies have shown that a very low-fat, plant-based diet in combination with daily exercise and stress-reduction techniques can reverse the progression of heart disease (the buildup of plaque on artery walls). The best plan, however, is to prevent heart disease from developing in the first place.

RESEARCH HIGHLIGHT
In the Male Health Professionals Study, the heart-protective effect achieved by consuming alpha-linolenic acid (a type of omega-3 fat found in canola oil, flaxseed and walnuts) was even more significant than reducing saturated fat in the diet. Saturated fats, often referred to as "bad" fats, come mostly from higher fat milk and meat products.

- Alpha-linolenic acid helps your heart to keep a strong and regular beat. A major cause of heart attacks is an irregular or chaotic beating of the heart that ultimately causes it to stop beating.

- Alpha-linolenic acid can be converted (to some extent) in the body from the plant form of omega-3 fats to the fish form of omega-3 fats (referred to as EPA/DPA). The fish form of omega-3 fats provides additional benefits, including reducing your risk of blood clots (often the first step in a heart attack), some cancers, arthritis, depression and more (read the Fantastic Fish chapter for all the details).

Limit the Amount of Omega-6 Fat You Eat

Another good reason to choose canola oil is that it contains almost equal amounts of omega-3 and omega-6 fats. In comparison, corn oil, sunflower oil, safflower oil and soybean oil (and all the products made with them, such as margarine or salad dressings) contain significantly more of the omega-6 fats. Much of the meat we eat is also rich in omega-6 fats (as well as saturated fats) as a result of the type of diet most animals are fed.

Why do we need to limit our intake of omega-6 fats? Evidence suggests that the diet of early humans—and the one for which our genetic make-up was programmed—contained equal amounts of these fats. Today it appears that many of us may be getting significantly more of the omega-6 fats than the omega-3 fats. Preliminary research suggests that the relative balance of these fats may be important for the prevention of disease. For example, a balanced intake of omega-6 and omega-3 fats appears to inhibit the development of some cancers. In addition, too much omega-6 fat in your diet prevents your body from converting alpha-linolenic acid (the plant form of omega-3 fats) to EPA/DHA (the very beneficial fish form).

Monounsaturated Fats Get Two Thumbs Up

While it's important to have a balanced intake of omega-3 and omega-6 fats (which are both types of polyunsaturated fat), the majority of the fat you consume should be monounsaturated. Canola oil meets this criterion also. It contains primarily monounsaturated fat. Monounsaturated fats help reduce your risk of heart disease by

- lowering LDL cholesterol (the bad kind that causes plaque to build up on artery walls) in your blood

- maintaining a healthy level of HDL cholesterol (the good kind that carries cholesterol out of the blood and back to the liver for disposal) in your blood

- helping lower triglycerides and certain lipo-proteins in your blood that are associated with heart disease when elevated

Monounsaturated fats may also help reduce your risk of some cancers, such as breast cancer, by helping prevent the development and spread of cancerous cells. Lastly, monounsaturated fats may help reduce your risk of diabetes by improving your sensitivity to insulin, thereby helping you maintain healthy blood sugar levels.

Olive Oil's Winning Formula

The traditional Mediterranean diet, rich in olive oil, is associated with low rates of disease and long life. The Ultimate Healthy Eating Plan recommends extra virgin olive oil. Here's why:

Proven Track Record

Olive oil, similar to canola oil, is very rich in monounsaturated fat and is also low in the omega-6 fats. As previously discussed, getting more monounsaturated fat in your diet, while limiting the amount of omega-6 fat you consume, appears to be important for reducing your risk of disease. Olive oil also has a proven track record. In the traditional Mediterranean diet, it is the primary source of fat. This diet is linked to a remarkable variety of health benefits including lower overall rates of cancer and heart disease.

Beneficial Plant Compounds Fight Disease

Olive oil, especially extra virgin olive oil, contains an abundance of beneficial plant compounds such as flavonoids, phenols and lignans. Many of these compounds appear to act as potent antioxidants in the body. They help fight disease by

- reducing the buildup of plaque on artery walls and preventing blood clots from forming

olive oil

RESEARCH HIGHLIGHT
Research from Stockholm involving over 60,000 women found that those who consumed the highest proportion of monounsaturated fats had the lowest risk of breast cancer.

TRUE OR FALSE?
The amount of cholesterol in the food you eat is the major factor that raises your blood cholesterol. False Eating too much saturated fat (high-fat milk and meat products) and hydrogenated fats (deep-fried fast foods, hard margarine and many processed foods) is what is most harmful to blood cho-lesterol levels.

RESEARCH HIGHLIGHT
In a recent study from southern Greece, those with the lowest lifetime consumption of extra virgin olive oil were over twice as likely to develop rheumatoid arthritis as compared to those with the highest intake.

- inhibiting the development and spread of cancerous cells, especially for breast and colon cancer

- helping maintain a healthy blood pressure by keeping artery walls flexible and open

The Margarine/Butter Debate

The Ultimate Healthy Eating Plan recommends a soft-tub, nonhydrogenated margarine that is low in saturated fat and made primarily with canola or olive oil (or both). Here's why:

Margarine Really Is Better Than Butter

Research clearly supports that a soft-tub, non-hydrogenated margarine can significantly decrease the LDL ("bad") cholesterol in your blood, while butter does just the opposite. A good margarine contains primarily healthy-for-you fats, while butter is a major source of saturated fat. For healthy blood cholesterol levels, it's important to limit your intake of saturated fats—the fats that are found primarily in high-fat milk and meat products. Another good reason to choose margarine over butter is it's an important source of vitamin E—another key player in the game of good health.

Hydrogenated Fats Are Nasty

It's important to choose a nonhydrogenated margarine, as opposed to a hard stick margarine, in order to minimize the hydrogenated fats (also called trans fats) in your diet. Hydrogenation (the adding of hydrogen) is a process used to turn a vegetable oil into a spreadable product. Hydrogenated vegetable oils are also used to improve the shelf life and stability of most processed foods (and I mean most!). Most donut shops and fast-food restaurants also use hydrogenated vegetable oils for their deep-frying. These fats can be nasty—especially if you consume a lot of them. They can harm your health by

- increasing the LDL ("bad") cholesterol in your blood

- decreasing the HDL ("good") cholesterol in your blood

- decreasing the elasticity or flexibility of blood vessel walls

- decreasing insulin sensitivity, thereby promoting unhealthy blood sugar levels

- preventing your body from converting the plant form of omega-3 fats (alpha-linolenic acid) into the beneficial fish form of omega-3 fats (EPA/DHA)

margarine

GOOD ADVICE

If you already suffer from heart disease or high blood cholesterol you should consider using a margarine, such as Becel Pro-Active, that contains added plant sterols. These plant compounds can lower blood cholesterol levels by 10% or more. They work by inhibiting the absorption of cholesterol from the small intestine.

RESEARCH HIGHLIGHT

In a study from the Texas Southwestern Medical Center involving 46 families, switching from butter to a soft-tub margarine was found to decrease LDL ("bad") cholesterol in the blood by an average of 11% for adults and 9% for children. Have you made the switch?

GOOD ADVICE

Oils in their natural states are an even better option than soft margarine. For example, instead of spreading your bread with margarine, simply dip it in a small amount of spiced olive or canola oil.

Bottom line: for good health get hydrogenated fats
out of your diet!

How Low Should You Go?

The Ultimate Healthy Eating Plan recommends enjoying
"healthy fats," but it also suggests still keeping the
overall fat content of your diet low.

The seven-day meal plans provided in the second
part of this book contain on average about 25% of
calories from fat. That is no more than about 50 to
60 grams of fat daily (based on 1800 to 2200
calorie levels). To some people, this sounds like a
lot of fat. However, fat grams add up quickly—
especially when you make foods like olive oil,
canola oil and nuts a regular part of your diet.
Here are some reasons to limit the overall fat
content of your diet:

Calorie Dense, But You're Still Hungry

Diets high in fat are high in calories, because fat
contains more than twice as many calories as protein
or carbohydrate. This would be fine if you felt so
satisfied after eating higher fat foods that you ate
less of other foods. Research suggests otherwise.
Most people tend to feel more satisfied (full) after
eating a meal containing protein and carbohydrate
(especially fiber-rich carbohydrates) as compared

hydrogenated fats

RESEARCH HIGHLIGHT
In the Nurses' Health Study,
involving over 80,000 women,
those women who consumed
the most hydrogenated fats
were 50% more likely to develop
heart disease and almost 40%
more likely to develop diabetes.

GOOD ADVICE
Watch out for food labels that
say "made with 100% vegetable
oil shortening." As soon as you
see the word "shortening," you
know the product contains
unhealthy hydrogenated or
trans fats.

RESEARCH HIGHLIGHT
Based on a review of 10
European countries, rates of
asthma and allergies among
teenagers were highest in
places where people ate the
most hydrogenated fats from
processed foods.

to a meal high in fat. (Think about it. How full do you feel after eating a bag of potato chips?)

The Fat You Eat Is the Fat You Wear

Your body is more efficient at storing calories from fat than storing calories from protein or carbohydrate. Therefore, even if you keep the total number of calories in your diet the same, you'll gain more body fat when you eat a higher fat diet.

Heart Attack Caused by Last Fatty Meal

Research suggests that two hours after eating a heavy, high-fat meal your risk of a heart attack quadruples. A high-fat meal causes a temporary increase in fatty particles that can build up on artery walls and also increase your risk of blood clots.

Your Daily Fat Quota

The Ultimate Healthy Eating Plan recommends consuming about 3 to 6 servings of added fats each day.

This amount includes the canola oil or extra virgin olive oil you use in cooking or drizzle on foods like tomatoes or bread. It also includes margarine, salad dressings, mayonnaise or other high-fat spreads.

Most women should choose the lower number of fat servings, and active men the higher number. Most other males can choose somewhere in between. These guidelines apply throughout the rest of the book to all ranges of recommended servings (with the exception of vegetables and fruit—everyone can eat more of those).

Things to Remember

Be sure to make or buy products such as margarine, salad dressing and mayonnaise that are made primarily with extra virgin olive oil or canola oil (or both!). Buy light or low-fat salad dressings and mayonnaise that contain about 3 to 4 grams of fat per serving. Do not buy fat-free versions of these products.

ONE FAT SERVING	1 tsp (5 mL) extra virgin olive oil or canola oil
	1 tsp (5 mL) nonhydrogenated margarine
	1 tbsp (15 mL) light or low-fat mayonnaise
	1 tbsp (15 mL) light or low-fat salad dressing
EXCEPTIONS TO THE 3 TO 6 SERVINGS RULE	consume 1 less serving of added fats on the days you have soy nuts
	consume 2 less servings of added fats on the days you have a full serving (2 tbsp / 25 mL) of peanut butter
	consume an extra serving of fat on the days you don't have nuts of any kind
	count 8 large olives as 1 serving of fat or one-quarter avocado as 2 servings of fat
	P.S. This is not as complicated as it may seem. In Part II, "Putting It All Together," we present four different seven-day meal plans to show you exactly how it's done.

THE ULTIMATE HEALTHY EATING PLAN

Enjoy 3 to 6 servings daily of canola oil, extra virgin olive oil or products made with these oils, such as soft, nonhydrogenated margarine, salad dressing and mayonnaise. Limit your intake of saturated fats found in higher fat meat and milk products. Minimize your intake of hydrogenated fats found in hard margarine, many processed foods and deep-fried fast foods.

PHENOMENAL
VEGETABLES AND FRUIT

THE OBJECTIVES OF THE ULTIMATE HEALTHY EATING PLAN ARE TO REDUCE YOUR RISK OF DISEASE BY

optimizing

vegetables and fruits overall | dark green, orange, and red vegetables and fruit | cruciferous vegetables | antioxidant-rich vegetables and fruit | tomatoes and tomato-based foods

DISEASE PROTECTION AT ITS BEST

Right now I want to jump up and down and scream and shout, just to make sure you're paying attention. (Here I go—jump, jump, jump. "Hey you, listen up. Pay attention. This is really important!") The reason for my enthusiasm is that I know you've heard this before—many times. My guess, however, is that as many times as you've heard it, you may still underestimate its value.

The message is this: eat your vegetables and fruit—lots of them. Eat them in the morning, eat them in the afternoon, eat them in the evening—eat them all day long (there's a song here somewhere). The research is strong and it's consistent. To significantly reduce your risk of cancer, heart disease, stroke, cataracts and more, vegetables and fruit are absolutely essential.

Disease-Fighting Powerhouses

What is it in vegetables and fruit that make them so powerful in the fight against disease? Vegetables and fruit contain a complex mix of health-protective vitamins, minerals and fiber, along with literally hundreds of beneficial plant compounds (also referred to as phytochemicals). This unique package of nutrients and plant compounds creates a disease-fighting environment in your body.

Antioxidant Protection

Vegetables and fruit protect your body from the damage caused by dangerous compounds called free radicals. We all have free radicals in our bodies. Every time your body uses oxygen, free radicals are produced. Infection or disease, as well as exposure to cigarette smoke or pollution, can also increase free-radical production.

Free radicals are nasty and can rapidly attack various cells in your body. For example, they can damage the LDL ("bad") cholesterol in your blood. When LDL becomes damaged, it's much

---

RESEARCH HIGHLIGHT
A review by 15 of the world's leading researchers in diet and cancer of over 4500 studies put vegetables and fruit at the top of the list of the foods most likely to reduce the risk of cancer.

QUESTION OF THE DAY
"Is it better to eat vegetables raw or cooked?" A combination of both raw and cooked veggies is best. Some nutrients, such as beta-carotene in carrots and lycopene in tomatoes, become more available to the body when foods are cooked. Cooking, however, can result in the loss of important water-soluble vitamins, like vitamin C, as well as other valuable plant compounds. When you do cook, use as little water as possible (soup is an exception since you consume the water) and cook veggies just until tender, but still crisp. Steaming, microwaving or stir-frying are all recommended cooking methods.

more likely to cause a buildup of plaque or fatty deposits on artery walls. Free radicals can also damage your DNA—the blueprint your cells use to reproduce. Damage to DNA is thought to be an essential step in the development of cancer. This is where antioxidants come in. They neutralize cell-damaging free radicals, putting them out of business. Vegetables and fruit are particularly rich sources of antioxidants such as vitamin C, beta-carotene and lycopene. Many of the hundreds of plant compounds found in vegetables and fruit also act as antioxidants in your body. Bottom line: to protect yourself from disease caused by free radicals, eat your vegetables and fruit.

Beyond Antioxidants

Other ways that compounds in vegetables and fruit protect against disease are by

- helping prevent the formation of blood clots that often cause a heart attack or stroke

- lowering LDL ("bad") cholesterol that promotes the buildup of plaque on artery walls

- helping maintain the health of blood vessel walls, including a healthy blood pressure

- stimulating the immune system, which plays a central role in disease protection

- influencing important enzymes in the body that help prevent, block or suppress the development of cancer

- protecting the retina of the eye and thereby reducing the risk of cataracts and macular degeneration (two of the most common causes of adult blindness)

The Five-to-Ten-a-Day Equation

The Ultimate Healthy Eating Plan recommends 5 to 10 servings of vegetables and fruit each day.

For those of you who love math, here's how the equation goes. Eating 5 to 10 servings of vegetables and fruit every day equals a significantly lower risk of disease. It's a simple equation with a powerful result. If the only thing you changed in your diet right now was to eat at least 5 servings of vegetables and fruit each day, you could reduce your risk of both heart disease and cancer by about 20% to 30% (or more!). And while 5 servings is the minimum number to shoot for, getting more than that is even better. A cancer research center in Colorado, for example, found that women who increased fruit and vegetable consumption beyond 5 servings per day saw significant reductions in the type of free-radical damage associated with heart disease and cancer. In the DASH study (dietary approach to stop hypertension), consuming 8 to

fighting disease

RESEARCH HIGHLIGHT
Broccoli, cauliflower, cabbage, kale and Brussels sprouts all belong to the cruciferous family of vegetables. In a study involving almost 6000 women from Sweden, those women who ate the most cruciferous vegetables were 24% less likely to develop breast cancer.

RESEARCH HIGHLIGHT
Preliminary research suggests that eating more vegetables and fruit may help fight osteoporosis by slowing bone loss. Vegetables and fruit are important sources of vitamin K and magnesium in the diet, and both nutrients appear to play an important role in bone health.

RESEARCH HIGHLIGHT
Based on the Nurses' Health Study and the Health Professionals Follow-Up Study, those who ate the most vegetables and fruit (an average of 5 to 6 servings per day) had a 30% lower risk of stroke compared to those who ate the least. The risk of coronary heart disease was 20% lower. Moral of the story: eat your vegetables and fruit!

10 servings of vegetables and fruit each day—along with an overall healthy diet—was associated with decreases in blood pressure normally achieved only with medication. For those of you who think 5 to 10 servings sounds like a truckload of vegetables and fruit, let me assure you it's only a wheelbarrow full (just kidding!). It's easy to get your 5-to-10-a-day when you realize what 1 serving looks like.

Good, Better, Best . . .

Is there such thing as a good, better and best vegetable or fruit to eat? The most important thing for you to remember is to eat a wide variety of vegetables and fruit and to eat lots of them. Having said that, some vegetables and fruit appear to be better equipped to reduce your risk of disease.

Dark Green, Orange, and Red Rule

The Ultimate Healthy Eating Plan recommends that at least half your daily vegetable and fruit choices are dark green, orange or red.

When it comes to veggies and fruit, color is an excellent indication of disease-fighting potential. Generally speaking, veggies and fruit that are dark green, bright orange or red contain the highest

ONE SERVING VEGETABLES AND FRUIT	
	1 medium-size vegetable or fruit (for example, a medium-size apple, orange or carrot)
	1/2 cup (125 mL) raw, cooked or frozen vegetable or fruit (for example, a scoop of cooked peas or a small bowl of sliced peaches)
	1/2 cup (125 mL) juice (for example, a small glass of orange or tomato juice)
	1 cup (250 mL) salad (for example, a small side salad)
	1/4 cup (50 mL) dried fruit (for example, a medium-size handful of raisins)

quantities of valuable nutrients and beneficial plant compounds. Many brightly colored vegetables and fruit are rich in nutrients such as beta-carotene (as well as other carotenoids like lutein, zeaxanthin, lycopene and alpha-carotene), vitamin C and folate. It is the color of the inside of the vegetable or fruit that is most important. Cucumbers, for example, have a dark green skin but are pale on the inside. They don't rank as nutritional all-stars. This doesn't mean you should stop eating cucumbers—they still contain many plant compounds

veggies + fruit

QUESTION OF THE DAY
"Does a minimum of 5 servings of vegetables and fruit each day mean 5 servings of vegetables plus 5 servings of fruit?" No, it means a total of 5 servings. For example, 3 servings of vegetables plus 2 servings of fruit equals 5 servings.

QUESTION OF THE DAY
"I like fruit, but I'm not too keen on veggies. Can I get my 5 daily servings by eating just fruit?" Sorry, not a good plan. Different kinds of vegetables and fruit contain different kinds of beneficial plant compounds that help fight disease in different ways. For full disease

protection, you want to eat a wide variety of both veggies and fruit. For example, only the cruciferous vegetables, such as broccoli, contain the potent anticancer compound called sulforaphane.

that may be valuable to health. It does mean you should choose the following brightly colored vegetables and fruit more often:

Dark Green asparagus, broccoli, Brussels sprouts, green peppers, kiwi, leafy greens (like spinach and kale)

Orange apricots, cantaloupe, carrots, oranges, mango, papaya, pumpkin, squash, sweet potatoes

Red pink grapefruit, raspberries, red cabbage, red peppers, strawberries, tomatoes, watermelon

When in Doubt, Eat Broccoli

The Ultimate Healthy Eating Plan recommends eating cruciferous vegetables (broccoli, Brussels sprouts, bok choy, cabbage, cauliflower, collards, kale, rutabaga, turnips) at least three times per week—and ideally more.

My first book was called *When in doubt, eat broccoli.* I chose the title because broccoli truly is one of those foods your body thanks you for eating. Broccoli is a member of the cruciferous family. Many studies have singled out cruciferous vegetables as providing the greatest protection against disease—often at an intake of at least 3 or more servings per week. These vegetables contain potent anti-cancer compounds called indoles and isothiocyanates (sulforaphane is one of the best-known isothiocyanates). These compounds block enzymes involved in the initial stages of cancer development and help detoxify carcinogens (cancer-causing compounds) that have already been formed. Kale and broccoli rank highest in this group in terms of their overall nutrient contribution. In terms of cooking, research suggests that the anti-cancer compounds in cruciferous vegetables are more available to your body when these vegetables are eaten raw. Most important, don't boil them. The compounds are water-soluble and will be lost in the water. Steam, microwave or stir-fry instead.

Berries and Dried Fruit

The Ultimate Healthy Eating Plan recommends that you make berries and dried fruit a regular part of your diet.

Researchers from the General Mills lab in Minnesota recently analyzed the antioxidant activity of various vegetables and fruit. Here are the top ten results (number 1 scored the highest antioxidant activity):

1. dates
2. raisins
3. prunes
4. blackberries
5. raspberries

GOOD ADVICE

Popeye was right. Dark leafy greens like spinach are good for you! The darker the green, the greater the nutritional value and disease-fighting potential. For example, spinach contains about twice as much potassium and folate and almost 3 times as much vitamin A as romaine lettuce. There's an even greater difference when it comes to iceberg lettuce (barely green in color). Spinach contains over 3 times as much potassium and folate and 20 times as much vitamin A. Other great greens include kale, collards, swiss chard, turnip greens, mustard greens and beet greens.

QUESTION OF THE DAY

"Can food slow the aging process?" In an animal study from Tufts University, blueberries improved motor skills and reversed the short-term memory loss that comes with aging. A few more berries in your diet certainly can't hurt.

6. blueberries
7. strawberries
8. red plums
9. black plums
10. red grapes

The moral of the story: berries and dried fruit (which, by the way, make up a relatively small part of the average diet!) are antioxidant all-stars. Make an effort to include them in your diet more often. Because dried fruit is a concentrated source of calories, don't eat more than 1/4 to 1/2 cup (50 to 125 mL) each day. Vegetables that get good marks in terms of antioxidant status include red cabbage, garlic, kale, spinach, Brussels sprouts, beets and broccoli.

You Say Tomato, I Say Tomato

The Ultimate Healthy Eating Plan recommends that you make tomatoes or tomato-based foods (tomato juice, spaghetti sauce or tomato soup) a regular part of your diet.

More and more studies put the spotlight on tomatoes as an important food for optimal health. In a recent review of 72 studies, 57 of them showed a link between high intakes of tomatoes or levels of lycopene in the blood (the plant compound found primarily in tomatoes) and a lower risk of cancer. The research was strongest for cancers of the prostate, lung and stomach. Studies also support a link between tomatoes and heart health.

Lycopene, like beta-carotene, is a member of the carotenoid family. Of all the carotenoids, lycopene demonstrates the highest antioxidant activity. The lycopene in heat-processed products like spaghetti sauce, the tomato sauce used on pizza, or tomato juice is more available to the body than that found in raw tomatoes. Heat breaks down the cell walls of the tomato, freeing the lycopene that would normally pass through your digestive system. That's why you get almost the same amount of lycopene from eating a whole tomato as you do from a tablespoon of ketchup. This doesn't mean you should give up on raw tomatoes, it simply means you should include processed tomato products in your diet as well. One note of caution: most processed tomato products are very high in sodium. Limit your intake to about 1 or 2 servings per day and choose lower sodium brands where available.

How the Ultimate Healthy Eating Plan Puts the Advice into Action

If you're thinking, "how am I possibly going to eat 5 to 10 servings of vegetables and fruit each day and make sure I get the dark green, orange, and

GOOD ADVICE

Enjoy your apples. Although apples don't get high marks for their overall nutritional content, they are excellent sources of plant compounds called flavonoids. These compounds appear to act as powerful antioxidants in the body and are linked to lower rates of heart disease and cancer. To get the best health protection from apples, you must eat them with the skin on; that's where you'll find most of the disease-fighting flavonoids.

RESEARCH HIGHLIGHT

Diets high in plant compounds called lutein and zeaxanthin—found in dark green, orange and red vegetables and fruit—can help save your sight by reducing your risk of cataracts and age-related macular degeneration (an eye disease that can lead to blindness). Corn is also a particularly good source of these plant compounds.

GOOD ADVICE

There are two great reasons to use lots of onions, garlic, scallions, leeks and chives when preparing meals. First, these vegetables—all members of the allium family—contain important sulfur-containing compounds that may help reduce your risk of cancer and heart disease. Second, they add so much wonderful flavor to food, you can use less salt when cooking and lower your risk of high blood pressure.

red ones and the cruciferous ones and some berries or dried fruit and some tomato or tomato-based foods?", here are 12 tips to help you on your way.

1 Be a Planner
Once a week, take just a few minutes to plan your meals for the week. This simple task can make all the difference in the nutritional quality of your diet! Do your grocery shopping based on this plan, making sure you stock up on all the recommended veggies and fruit.

2 Eat Them All Day Long
Include at least 1 (and ideally more than 1) serving of vegetables or fruit with every meal. Then snack on them—during the morning, the afternoon and even in the evening. Don't worry, you will not turn into a rabbit. (You may feel like a rabbit, your friends may think you're a rabbit, but you will not be a rabbit.)

3 Liquid Nutrition
Start each day with a glass of orange juice. How easy is that! It falls into the "orange" category and a mere 1/2 cup (125 mL) counts as 1 serving. An easy way to get more tomato in your life is with tomato juice. Buy a large bottle for your fridge at home. Then stock up on the small cans that are perfect for an afternoon snack. Two things to

---

LYCOPENE CONTENT

(Lycopene is a plant compound linked to lower rates of disease.)

ketchup (1 tbsp/15 mL)	3 mg
raw tomato	4 mg
pink grapefruit	5 mg
tomato soup (1 cup/250 mL)	10 mg
watermelon (1 slice)	15 mg
tomato juice (1 cup/250 mL)	25 mg
spaghetti sauce (1/2 cup/125 mL)	28 mg

RESEARCH HIGHLIGHT
Folate (also called folic acid) is one more great reason to eat your dark green and orange vegetables and fruit. Studies suggest that the nutrient folate may significantly reduce the risk of heart disease by lowering levels of homocysteine (a byproduct of the body's breakdown of protein) in the blood. Homocysteine is believed to damage blood vessel walls and encourage the buildup of plaque on artery walls. Vitamin B12 (found in lean meats, fish, milk products, fortified soy milk) and B6 (found in whole grains, bananas, potatoes, fish, lean meats) are also important for healthy homocysteine levels.

broccoli

RESEARCH HIGHLIGHT
Researchers from Johns Hopkins University have found that broccoli sprouts have an amazingly high concentration of the cancer-fighting plant compound called sulforaphane—20 to 50 times more than mature broccoli. In animal studies, sulforaphane has brought about truly dramatic reductions in cancer risk. The downside? Raw sprouts of any kind can be a source of harmful bacteria. For this reason it is recommended that people who are more vulnerable to infection, including young children and older adults, avoid sprouts altogether.

P.S. Broccoli still contains considerably more fiber, vitamin C and vitamin A than broccoli sprouts.

RESEARCH HIGHLIGHT
Potassium, a nutrient found primarily in vegetables and fruit, is linked to a lower risk of high blood pressure and stroke.

RESEARCH HIGHLIGHT
People who eat lots of vegetables are more likely to maintain a healthy body weight.

remember when it comes to juice: First, fruit juice is lacking in fiber and is a concentrated source of calories. Enjoy no more than 1 to 2 servings each day. Second, since most vegetable juices are high in sodium, limit your intake also to 1 or 2 servings each day and choose lower sodium brands where available.

4 Don't Leave Home Without Them!

This tip makes all the difference between barely meeting and totally exceeding your minimum 5-a-day quota. It's simple. Never (and I mean never) leave your home without packing some portable vegetables or fruit in your knapsack, purse, brief-case or the glove compartment of your car. During the day, you're going to get hungry, guaranteed! Rather than playing vending-machine roulette or stopping at a convenience store that makes it convenient to eat poorly, reach for your own personal stash of veggies or fruit. Easy-to-carry options include apples, pears, bananas, mandarin oranges or clementines, canned fruit cups, baby carrots, cherry or grape tomatoes, dried fruits, grapes and juice paks. Even a kiwi can be portable; simply cut it in half ahead of time and when you get hungry at work just scoop it out with a spoon. Carrying a small pack of wet wipes with you is also a good idea. It makes cleanup a breeze.

5 Stuff Your Sandwich

Sandwiches are still the most popular item when it comes to lunch. Don't let your sandwich get lonely. Every time you make or order a sandwich, pile on the veggies or fruit. Sliced tomatoes, cucumbers and dark leafy greens are sandwich necessities. Strips of green or red peppers, roasted or raw, make nutritious, delicious sandwich stuffers. Bananas and peanut butter were meant to go together. Shredded carrots or finely chopped red or green peppers go great with tuna or salmon salad sandwich mixtures. Chopped fruit, like peaches, pears, apricots or apples, are wonderful with mix-tures of chicken or turkey salad. At restaurants, use salad bars to make nutritious veggie-filled sandwiches. When you can't put veggies or fruit in your sandwich, enjoy a few strips of carrot or red pepper on the side.

6 Buy Convenience

I can't tell you the number of people who now enjoy salad seven days a week, 365 days of the year (slight exaggeration), all because of prewashed and bagged salads. Simply tear them open, add dressing and eat. Be sure to buy the dark leafy greens! Other great time-saving products include baby car-rots, chopped veggies like broccoli and cauliflower, shredded veggies like cabbage, salad bar produce,

herbs and olive oil

GOOD ADVICE
Be generous with herbs and spices when cooking. Many are rich in beneficial plant com-pounds that may further reduce your risk of disease. They're also great flavor enhancers that make it easy to use less salt. The following herbs have been identified by the National Cancer Institute as possessing cancer-preventive properties: basil, mint, oregano, rosemary, sage, thyme, turmeric (often found in curry powder), ginger, anise, caraway, celery, chervil, cilantro, coriander, cumin, dill, fennel, parsley, tarragon.

RESEARCH HIGHLIGHT
Olive oil and tomatoes are a good combination. In a study from Ireland, eating tomato products with olive oil, but not with sunflower oil, resulted in better antioxidant activity in the blood.

sliced mushrooms, roasted red peppers (in a jar), and ready-made dips for veggies or fruit.

7 Make Room for Frozen and Canned

Who said that canned or frozen fruits and vegetables are not high-quality nutritional choices? On the contrary, these vegetables and fruit are harvested at the peak of ripeness and prepared for canning or freezing within hours of being picked. This process guarantees great nutrition as well as great taste. In contrast, fresh produce—especially during the winter months—can lose valuable nutrients during travel and storage time. For example, in one study, after one year, frozen spinach was found to retain more than twice the vitamin C of fresh spinach that had spent just seven days in refrigeration (both samples came from the same crop). One of the easiest ways to get more berries in your diet is to add frozen berries to smoothies or shakes. Two final words of advice about frozen and canned produce: buy frozen vegetables instead of canned to limit your salt intake and avoid frozen veggies with added sauces.

8 Order Right When Dining Out

Research shows that when dining out, most people eat less vegetables and fruit—especially when eating at fast-food restaurants. Here are some tips to prevent this from happening to you:

- Choose restaurants that serve vegetables and fruit (I know I can get a salad or baked potato at Wendy's).

- Enjoy a salad as an appetizer or even as a main course meal. Always ask for low-fat or light dressing on the side so you can control how much you eat.

- Ask whether the entrée comes with vegetables. If not, order extra veggies on the side. (Sorry, french fries don't count.)

- Supplement take-out dinners with vegetables and fruit from home. Microwaved veggies are fast and easy, and canned fruit like mandarin orange sections make a quick dessert.

9 Double Up

If you normally take one scoop of peas, take two. Instead of three spears of asparagus, have six. Skip the second helping of dessert, have a second helping of broccoli. It doesn't get any easier than this!

10 Dip It

Vegetables and dip—is there a more splendid combination? Vegetables were born to be dipped (most kids would agree!). Simply buy a creamy salad dressing for dipping (no fat-free allowed, lower fat or light is okay—we need those healthy fats) and go wild with carrot sticks, red pepper

fruit juice

QUESTION OF THE DAY

"What's the best type of fruit juice to drink?" That's a tough question. Orange juice gets high marks for its vitamin C and folate content, plus the fact you can buy it calcium-enriched. Several studies link citrus fruits, including oranges, to a lower risk of heart disease and cancer. As for purple grape juice (made from concord grapes), preliminary research gives it high marks for its antioxidant potential (three times higher than grapefruit, orange or apple juice) and for its ability to help your heart by dilating blood vessels and reducing the formation of blood clots. My advice? For most people orange juice should be the first priority. As further research unfolds about grape juice, it may deserve a more prominent place in your diet, especially if you suffer from heart disease. Most important, to limit calories, limit your intake of fruit juice to no more than 1 cup (250 mL) per day.

strips, broccoli and cauliflower florets and more. Fresh fruit, such as bananas, berries or orange sections, taste great dipped in either low-fat fruit-flavored yogurt or low-fat chocolate pudding.

11   Eliminate the Competition

The more cookies, chips and candy you have in your cupboards or your desk at work, the less likely you are to reach for vegetables or fruit (sad, but true). That's the reason it's critical to keep unhealthy but tempting goodies out of sight and out of reach. (Better yet, don't keep them around at all!) Then make it easy to see and reach for vegetables and fruit. Keep a bowl filled with fruit on your kitchen counter at home and on your desk at work. Your family and co-workers will thank you for it. Always keep baby carrots or cut-up veggies in your fridge. Make them the first thing you see when you (or your kids) open the fridge door.

12   Five-Star Recipes

Check out the seven-day meal plans in the second part of this book and be sure to make the incredibly nutritious, incredibly delicious, disease-fighting, fruit-and-veggie-filled recipes provided.

The Pesticide Question

Should you buy organic produce? Dr. Bruce Ames, a multiple award winner for cancer research from the University of California at Berkeley, states, "The amounts of pesticide residues ingested are so small relative to levels that have been shown to have toxicological effects, they are toxicologically implausible as health risks." The Environmental Protection Agency in the United States reports that while about one out of every three people who gets excessive exposure to the sun will develop cancer in their lifetime, only one out of every 100,000 people or less will develop cancer from human-made chemicals in foods, including pesticides. Lastly, research suggests that simple household preparation, like rinsing and scrubbing, can remove anywhere from 30% to almost 100% of residues. My thoughts? Buying organic is a fine choice, but you don't have to. Do make sure you rinse and scrub all fresh fruit and vegetables thoroughly under running water. Don't use soap. You may end up consuming soap residues rather than pesticide residues.

GOOD ADVICE
Increase your vegetable intake by snacking on baby carrots or other cut-up veggies when preparing dinner. It's an easy way to get more veggies in your life.

MORE GOOD ADVICE
Become famous for the wonderful fruit or veggie trays you bring to parties. Let everyone get healthy together!

THE ULTIMATE HEALTHY EATING PLAN

Enjoy 5 to 10 servings of vegetables and fruit each day—at least half of which are dark green, orange or red in color. Enjoy cruciferous vegetables like broccoli, kale or Brussels sprouts at least three times during the week and ideally more. Also make berries or dried fruits a regular part of your diet and regularly enjoy tomatoes and tomato-based foods.

WONDERFUL
WHOLE GRAINS

THE OBJECTIVES OF THE ULTIMATE HEALTHY EATING PLAN ARE TO REDUCE YOUR RISK OF DISEASE BY

optimizing

whole-grain foods | whole-grain cereals

limiting

refined grains

THE WHOLE-GRAIN QUESTION

Do you like bread? How about pasta? And cereal? Most people like grains. That's good. They're an important source of fuel for our bodies. The key question, however, is do you eat your grains whole? Do you eat whole-grain breads? Do you eat whole-wheat pasta? Do you eat whole-grain cereals, rice, bagels and tortillas? To significantly reduce your risk of heart disease, cancer, diabetes and more, your grains have got to be whole.

The Whole-Grain Story

All grains, whether from wheat, oats, rice, corn or other sources, are made up of three parts—the bran, the endosperm and the germ. Each part has a special contribution to make.

The bran, or outer layer, contains

- a rich assortment of minerals such as iron, copper, zinc, magnesium, manganese and selenium

- generous amounts of fiber

- large amounts of B vitamins such as thiamin, riboflavin, niacin and folic acid

- significant amounts of beneficial plant compounds (many of which appear to act as potent antioxidants in the body)

The endosperm, or middle layer, contains

- mostly protein and carbohydrates

QUESTION OF THE DAY

"I thought high carbohydrate diets were bad because they cause trigylcerides in your blood—a risk factor for heart disease—to go up. Is this true?" Studies suggest that a diet high in refined carbohydrates (processed cakes, cookies, snack foods, white bread) can increase blood triglyceride levels. A high carbohydrate diet that emphasizes whole grains, beans, vegetables and fruit, however, has a beneficial effect on triglyceride levels.

RESEARCH HIGHLIGHT

In the Nurses' Health Study, those women who ate the most whole grains as compared to those women who ate the least reduced their risk of heart disease by 25% and stroke by over 30%.

The germ, or inner core, contains

- significant amounts of vitamin E
- some minerals and B vitamins
- a variety of beneficial plant compounds

When grains are refined or milled to make white bread, white rice, pasta and most crackers, cookies and cakes, the nutrient-rich, plant-compound-rich bran and germ are discarded. Only the endosperm or middle layer of the grain is used. Most refined products are then enriched with iron and B vitamins (these nutrients are added back) to make up for some of the losses that take place during refining. What is not added back, however, are most of the minerals, the vitamin E, the fiber and the many valuable plant compounds—all of which play very important roles in optimizing health. Bottom line: for good health from grains, eat them whole.

Health Protection and Whole Grains

How do whole grains reduce your risk of heart disease, cancer, diabetes and more? Like vegetables and fruit, whole grains contain a very complex mix of disease-fighting vitamins, minerals, fiber and beneficial plant compounds. Here are just some of the ways they protect your health:

Create a Healthy Gut Environment

Whole grains are rich sources of fermentable carbohydrates, including fiber, resistant starch and oligosaccharides. A fermentable carbohydrate is one that resists digestion until it reaches your colon, where it serves as food for the bacteria there. During this fermentation process, health-protective substances (short chain fatty acids) are produced, which inhibit the growth of cancerous tumors in the gut.

Keeps Things Moving Along

People who eat lots of whole grains are much less likely to suffer from constipation. The fiber in whole grains increases stool bulk. This promotes quicker elimination of body wastes, reducing the amount of time the colon is exposed to potential cancer-causing substances. Whole grains also reduce the incidence of hemorrhoids and diverticular disease (pouches or pockets that form in the wall of the colon). It's been said that we spend about three years of our life in the bathroom. Shouldn't those years be as enjoyable as possible?

Down with Cholesterol

Whole grains decrease LDL ("bad") cholesterol levels, thereby reducing the buildup of plaque on artery walls. They also help maintain a healthy blood pressure and reduce injury to the blood vessel walls.

health protection

RESEARCH HIGHLIGHT
In the Iowa Women's Health Study, the risk of dying from any cause—including heart disease and cancer—was found to be significantly lower in women who ate more whole grains as compared to refined grains.

RESEARCH HIGHLIGHT
In a review of 51 studies, 46 linked whole grains to a lower risk of cancer. The link was especially strong for gastrointestinal cancers such as colon cancer.

RESEARCH HIGHLIGHT
In the Nurses' Health Study, those women who ate the most whole grains had an almost 40% lower risk of developing diabetes than those who ate the least. Women who ate the most refined grains and the least whole grains had an almost 60% greater risk of developing diabetes.

Antioxidant Protection

Whole grains are a rich source of nutrients (vitamin E and selenium) and plant compounds (phenolic acids, phytic acid and lignans) that appear to act as potent antioxidants in the body. These nutrients and plant compounds are found primarily in the bran and germ. They help protect your body cells from the damage caused by free radicals, which can lead to heart disease and cancer.

Good for Blood Sugar

Whole grains contain a variety of substances, such as fiber, magnesium and various plant compounds, that appear to reduce the risk of diabetes by improving sensitivity to insulin and helping maintain healthy blood sugar levels.

Going for Grains

The Ultimate Healthy Eating Plan recommends 5 to 12 servings of grain products each day. Most, and ideally all, of the servings should be whole grain. Most women and anyone watching their waistline should consume closer to 5 servings per day. A very active male may eat closer to 12 servings.

ONE SERVING OF WHOLE GRAINS (INCLUDING WHOLE-WHEAT)	
	1 slice whole-grain bread
	1/2 whole-grain hamburger bun
	1/2 whole-grain English muffin
	1/2 whole-grain small bagel
	1/2 of a 6-inch (15-cm) whole-grain pita bread
	1 (6-inch/15-cm) whole-grain tortilla
	1/2 cup (125 mL) brown rice
	1/2 cup (125 mL) whole-wheat pasta
	1/2 cup (125 mL) whole-wheat couscous
	1 oz (30 g) whole-grain ready-to-eat cereal
	that's about 3/4 to 1 cup (175 to 250 mL) of most cereals; the cereal box label indicates what 1 oz (30 g) represents
	3/4 cup (175 mL) whole-grain, cooked cereal
	3 to 4 small whole-grain crackers
	1 (4-inch/10-cm) whole-grain pancake
	1 small whole-grain muffin

QUESTION OF THE DAY
"Aren't foods like bread and pasta fattening?" Research suggests otherwise, especially when it comes to whole grains. Studies have found that people who eat more whole grains are more likely to maintain a healthy body weight.

QUESTION OF THE DAY
"How much oatmeal do I need to eat each day to lower the amount of cholesterol in my blood?" A review of 10 studies concluded that the daily consumption of 3 grams of soluble fiber from oat products results in lower blood cholesterol levels. To get that amount of soluble fiber you would need to eat 1 1/2 cups (375 mL) cooked oatmeal, three packets instant oatmeal, or 3 cups (750 mL) of Cheerios.

QUESTION OF THE DAY
"Is instant oatmeal considered whole grain?" Steel-cut oats, old-fashioned oats, quick-cooking oats, rolled oats and instant oatmeal are all whole-grain oat products—all three parts of the grain remain after milling.

Other Grains

Many people have difficulty identifying whether or not a product is whole grain. In addition to the products listed above, the grains listed below are considered whole. These grains may be cooked on their own but are often found in soups, salads, cereals, breads or side dishes. (We give you some great ideas on how to use them in the recipe section of this book.)

- amaranth
- barley
- buckwheat
- bulgar
- graham flour
- kamut
- millet
- quinoa
- spelt
- triticale
- wheat berries

Make it a habit to enjoy a wide variety of whole-grain products. Quinoa, for example, has a chewy texture and a nutty taste. It is so rich in nutrients that some food experts refer to it as the super-grain of the future (try our Quinoa Pilaf on page 185).

Build a Beautiful Bowl

The Ultimate Healthy Eating Plan recommends that you start most days with a bowl of whole-grain cereal.

Regular cereal eaters are more likely to meet their daily nutrient requirements. The right cereal significantly boosts your fiber intake for the day. The average antioxidant activity of many whole-grain cereals is equal to or exceeds many vegetables or fruits. Cereal served with milk helps contribute to your daily requirement for calcium and vitamin D. Cereal is fast and fits easily into life in the fast lane.

Top Seven Steps for Building a Beautiful Bowl of Cereal
(total time to build and eat: 10 to 15 minutes max)

1 Start with 3/4 to 1 cup (175 to 250 mL) of whole-grain cereal, such as oatmeal (instant or regular), Cheerios, Shreddies, Weetabix, Shredded Wheat, Mini-Wheats, Raisin Bran or Post Fruit & Fibre. It should contain a minimum of 2 grams of fiber per serving and ideally more. Women (especially prior to menopause) should choose cereals that are iron enriched (regular oatmeal and Shredded Wheat, for example, are not).

2 Add about 1/4 to 1/2 cup (50 to 125 mL) of a very high fiber cereal such as All-Bran, Bran

glycemic index

QUESTION OF THE DAY

"I've heard it's not good to eat foods that are high on the glycemic index. What types of foods should I avoid?" The glycemic index is a measure of how fast a particular food is likely to raise your blood sugar. Recent studies suggest that people who eat a lot of foods with a high glycemic index may increase their risk of heart disease, diabetes, colon cancer and obesity. Generally, less refined, whole-grain products, especially barley and oats, have a lower glycemic index. Most important advice? Enjoy a wide variety of whole grains, vegetables, fruit and beans (all sources of carbohydrates). Eat smaller, more frequent meals. Limit the amount of highly processed, refined grains you eat. Maintain a healthy weight and exercise regularly.

Buds or Fibre 1. This is especially important if the cereal you chose in step 1 contains less than 4 grams of fiber per serving. This addition gives you another 5 to 10 grams or more of fiber.

3 Sprinkle with 1 tablespoon (15 mL) of ground flaxseed (more details in the Fabulous Flax chapter).

4 Add 1/2 cup (125 mL) fresh fruit such as blueberries or 1/2 banana or 1/4 cup (50 mL) dried fruit like raisins.

5 Pour on skim or 1% milk.

6 What about sugar? My rule for sugar is this: use it in small quantities to increase your enjoyment of healthy foods. For example, enjoy a sprinkle of sugar on cereal, enjoy jam on whole-grain toast or have syrup with your whole-grain pancakes.

7 Last but not least, don't forget to enjoy your cereal with a glass of fruit juice—the vitamin C will help you absorb more iron from the cereal.

Keep in mind that you don't have to limit your cereal eating to just breakfast. If you're tired and don't feel like cooking, don't go for fast-food— enjoy a quick and tasty bowl of cereal (have two bowls if you're still hungry). It's also a great after-school snack for kids. If your kids like presweetened cereals, make sure to buy whole-grain options like Quaker Instant Oatmeal or Golden Honey Shreddies.

Five More Great Ways to Add Whole Grains to Your Day

Here are five more tips to assist you in your quest for whole grains:

1 Muffin Madness

On the weekend, make a double batch of home-made whole-grain muffins. (If you own only one muffin baking pan, now's the time to buy a second. Your time is precious.) Keep the muffins in an air-tight container in the fridge or freeze them in individual baggies. Eat them throughout the week. They make great snacks at home and at work. For optimum taste, warm them in the microwave just before eating. The muffin recipes in this book are truly outstanding and loaded with good stuff!

2 Mama Mia

Enjoy whole-wheat pasta with a tomato-based sauce on a regular basis. Try Mairlyn's Amazing Tomato Sauce (page 193) or buy a store-bought sauce. Look for brands that contain less salt. Stay away from alfredo or cream-type sauces. They're

whole-grain snacks

GOOD ADVICE
When buying breads or crackers, check the ingredient list. Choose products made with only "whole-grain" or "whole-wheat" flours. Some multigrain or seven-grain breads, for example, list "wheat flour" as the first ingredient—another way of saying white refined flour. Many tortillas, pita breads and bagels are made with a combination of whole grains and refined grains. Go for 100% whole grain or whole wheat whenever possible.

GOOD ADVICE
Looking for a whole-grain snack? Popcorn and most low-fat, baked tortilla chips are whole grain. Go easy on the toppings when it comes to popcorn. Enjoy baked tortilla chips with generous amounts of tomato-rich salsa.

called "heart attack on a plate" for good reason. Pesto sauces made with olive oil are acceptable, but watch your serving size since they're a very concentrated source of fat and calories.

3 Pancakes and French Toast for Dinner

Try the whole-grain pancakes and french toast recipes in this book. Serve them for dinner when you don't have time to prepare a more elaborate meal. (My kids love getting pancakes for dinner—especially if I throw in a few chocolate chips.) Go easy on the toppings. Try the "light" syrups; they contain about half the calories of regular syrup and still taste great.

4 Beautiful Brown Rice

Every time you make a batch of brown rice, double it. Cooked rice stores up to seven days in the fridge. Simply reheat it with a little extra water in the microwave or on the stove for meals later in the week. Try our Brown Rice with Dried Cranberries and Orange (page 180). It's an easy way to make brown rice taste even better.

5 Did You Say Cookies?

Can you believe it? We included two whole-grain cookie recipes in this book for all the diehard cookie lovers. Make them just once in a while, and eat only 1 or 2 cookies at a time (share them with neighbors and friends if you have to). They put your average store-bought cookie to shame. They're also great as an occasional school lunch-box treat—especially when your kids complain that all the other kids get to bring chips or candy to school. Another way to satisfy a craving for something sweet is to enjoy a piece of whole-grain toast with some honey or jam.

Pass on the White Bread

The Ultimate Healthy Eating Plan recommends that you limit your intake of refined grains to about 1 to 2 servings per day. However, ideally all your choices should be whole grain.

Not only does research indicate that whole grains protect our health, it also tells us that refined grains may be harmful to health—especially for people who are overweight or inactive. People who eat lots of refined grains may be more likely to suffer from diabetes, heart disease and possibly some cancers. Limit your intake of

- white bread, rolls, buns, English muffins, tortillas, bagels, biscuits, pita bread

- refined pasta

- white rice

bread & cereal

QUESTION OF THE DAY

"Is rye bread or pumpernickel bread considered whole grain?" No. Many people mistakenly believe that if the bread is dark in color it must be whole grain. Although some whole-grain rye breads are available, most pumpernickel and rye products are made mostly with white flour and caramel or other added coloring.

GOOD ADVICE

Most but not all cereals are enriched with iron. Most women, especially prior to menopause, do not get enough iron in their diets. It's important for them to choose cereals that are both whole grain and iron enriched. Shredded Wheat, for example, is whole grain, but not iron enriched (Kellogg's Mini-Wheats are). Most regular oatmeal is not enriched, but instant oatmeal is.

QUESTION OF THE DAY

"Is it better to buy breads that have been stone-ground?" Stone-ground refers to a technique for grinding grains. It usually means that the grain is coarser. Some research indicates that grains with a larger particle size may help reduce the risk of heart disease. Most important, if you buy stone-ground bread, make sure it's whole grain or whole wheat.

- refined-grain breakfast cereals (there are lots of them out there, including many kids' cereals)

- most muffins, cakes, cookies, brownies, donuts and other desserts

- most pancakes and waffles

- most crackers

- pizza crust

Limiting your intake of refined grains can be particularly difficult if you dine out frequently. Many restaurants still serve primarily white bread or rolls. Whole-wheat pasta or pizza made with a whole-grain crust is pretty much nonexistent on the restaurant scene. Do your best by limiting your portion sizes and asking for whole-grain options where possible.

RESEARCH HIGHLIGHT
In the Seven Countries Study a daily increase of 10 grams of fiber was associated with a 33% lower risk of dying from colon cancer. Adults should aim to get 25 to 35 grams of fiber each day. For children use the following formula: age + 5 (for example, a child of age 7 needs 12 grams of fiber daily).

QUESTION OF THE DAY
"What is psyllium?" It has been called the single most effective dietary ingredient for lowering blood cholesterol. It is a natural grain that has eight times as much cholesterol-lowering, soluble fiber as oat bran. It is found in Kellogg's All-Bran Buds cereal, as well as laxatives such as Metamucil. People with high blood cholesterol levels or problems with regularity should consider making it a regular part of their diet. For the rest of us, eating a wide variety of whole-grain products is what's most important.

LOOKING-GOOD,
LOW-FAT MILK PRODUCTS

THE OBJECTIVES OF THE ULTIMATE HEALTHY EATING PLAN ARE TO REDUCE YOUR RISK OF DISEASE BY

optimizing

lower fat milk products | calcium

| vitamin D

MILK MAKES SENSE

How would you like to lower your risk of osteoporosis, high blood pressure and colon cancer and get a concentrated hit of important vitamins and minerals in the process? It has been an exciting time for research into milk products and the nutrients they contain. There are lots of good reasons to make them a regular part of your diet.

Building Beautiful Bones

Imagine picking up a bag of groceries and breaking your wrist, getting a hug from your spouse and breaking your ribs, or losing 4 inches (10 cm) in height because the bones in your spine are so weak they start to collapse. This is osteoporosis—the disease of fragile or brittle bones. While many people have heard of it, most don't realize how devastating and debilitating it can be. It often leads to chronic disabling pain (especially fractures of the spine) and has a profound impact on quality of life (fear, anxiety, depression and loss of mobility are frequently reported in women with osteoporosis).

The good news? Calcium makes a difference. Scientific evidence is overwhelming that lifelong calcium intake is one of the most significant factors determining your risk of an osteoporotic fracture. Calcium is key for both building and maintaining strong bones. The easiest and most efficient way to get calcium is with milk products.

RESEARCH HIGHLIGHT
It's never too late to get more calcium and vitamin D in your diet. In a three-year study involving over 3000 older women living in nursing homes (many over 80 years of age), increasing calcium by 1200 mg and vitamin D by 800 IU per day reduced fracture rates by almost 25%.

GOOD ADVICE
If you have kids, make sure they're active and consuming a calcium-rich diet. Think of their bones as a bank account. Making regular deposits of calcium during childhood and adolescence helps them build the strongest bones possible. Strong bones are better equipped to handle the withdrawals that occur later in life. More than 90% of bone mass is attained before 20 years of age.

RESEARCH HIGHLIGHT
Women in an osteoporosis prevention study were given 1000 mg of calcium daily either as a supplement (pill) or from milk products. The women getting their calcium from milk products improved their intake not only of calcium but of 11 other nutrients as well. Bottom line: for more nutrition, milk products make sense.

More Than Just Calcium

Most people think "calcium" when they think "milk." And yet what about vitamin D, vitamin B12, riboflavin, phosphorus, vitamin A, potassium, magnesium, protein, vitamin B6, thiamin and zinc? These nutrients are also found in milk products, many of them in good supply. That's the reason a diet lacking in milk products is often a poor diet, not just in respect to calcium but for many other nutrients as well. Meeting overall nutritional requirements is essential not only for good health but also for optimal disease prevention.

The Sunshine Vitamin

Imagine having the finest bricks in the land to build a strong, beautiful house, yet not being able to use them. Such is the story of calcium and vitamin D. While calcium is the essential, all-star bone-building material, vitamin D is necessary for the effective absorption of calcium from your diet. Without vitamin D, you absorb about 50% less calcium. Once calcium is absorbed, vitamin D also plays a role in depositing the calcium in your bones and teeth. How do you get vitamin D? Ten to 15 minutes of sunlight on your arms and face two to three times a week is one way. (Vitamin D is made in your body when sunlight strikes your skin.) However, in Canada and the northern United States, you could sit naked on your roof from mid-October to mid-April and still not produce enough! In summer, thanks to the regular use of sunscreens, the production of vitamin D is also minimal. Lastly, your body's ability to produce vitamin D decreases significantly with age.

That's why milk is so important. Very few foods are naturally good sources of vitamin D (higher fat fish like salmon are an exception). That's why in Canada and the United States vitamin D is added to milk (it's not added to cheese, yogurt or ice cream) and added in smaller quantities to margarine. It's also added to most soy beverages. In addition to fighting osteoporosis, vitamin D may also help reduce your risk of some cancers—especially breast, prostate and colon cancer—and possibly play a role in the treatment of arthritis and depression.

Beyond Osteoporosis

Although milk products have long been associated with the prevention of osteoporosis, more recent research suggests they may also play an important role in helping reduce your risk of colon cancer and high blood pressure.

Lower Risk of Colon Cancer

Research indicates that people with higher intakes

Calcium & Vitamin D

RESEARCH HIGHLIGHT
Research suggests that the diet of early humans—and for which our genetic make-up was programmed—was high in both calcium and vitamin D (much of the vitamin D came from daily exposure to the sun).

RESEARCH HIGHLIGHT
News alert: National calcium deficit. Research consistently shows that many people—especially women, teenaged girls and seniors—are not meeting recommended intakes for calcium. In a recent study involving over 500 women across Canada, only 12% were meeting the recommended daily intake of 1000 mg of calcium. Are you getting enough?

GOOD ADVICE
Buy calcium-enriched milk like Trucalcium made by Neilson. It contains 33% more calcium than regular milk.

of calcium and vitamin D are less likely to develop cancer of the colon. Calcium appears to bind with compounds (fatty acids and bile salts) that are potentially toxic to the colon. Calcium and vitamin D also appear to reduce the development and spread of cancerous cells. Milk products appear to provide better protection than does taking calcium in the form of a supplement.

Lower Risk of High Blood Pressure

The DASH study (dietary approach to stop hypertension) looked at the effects of diet on blood pressure. The greatest reductions in blood pressure were seen with a diet rich in vegetables and fruit (8 to 10 servings) and low-fat milk products (about 3 servings). The level of blood pressure reduction achieved was far greater than that observed in any prior nutritional study of blood pressure regulation. The combination of vegetables, fruit and milk products was most important (fruits and vegetables alone lowered blood pressure but not by nearly as much as when combined with milk products). Calcium is thought to be a key player in blood pressure regulation. It helps reduce blood pressure by relaxing and dilating (widening) the artery walls.

But I Eat Lots of Broccoli . . .

How easy is it to meet your daily calcium requirement from foods other than milk products? It's not! Let's take broccoli. It's often touted as a good source of calcium that's absorbed well by the body. While broccoli is a wonderful food and I hope you enjoy it often, do you eat 7 cups (1.75 L) daily? That's how much is required to replace the calcium in 3 servings of milk products. Kale and bok choy are other vegetables that contain good quantities of easily absorbed calcium, but again these foods are not featured on most people's daily menus. Spinach contains calcium, but your body can't use most of it because it's bound to plant compounds called oxalates. Much of the calcium in most beans is also unavailable. And what about nutrients like vitamin D or vitamin B12? You won't get them by eating foods like broccoli or beans.

There is only one food that is nutritionally similar to cow's milk and that is fortified soy milk (with added nutrients like calcium, vitamin D, riboflavin and vitamin B12). Three servings (1 serving = 1 cup / 250 mL) of cow's milk each day can be replaced by 3 servings of fortified soy milk (also called soy beverage). For most people, however, a diet that includes both dairy products and soy (see Sensational Soy chapter for more details) provides the best mix of taste, variety and disease prevention.

RESEARCH HIGHLIGHT

A study of more than 2500 postmenopausal women indicated that women with low bone density (which may lead to osteoporosis) are at a significantly greater risk of gum disease, which is the major cause of tooth loss in those over the age of 35. Calcium is thought to contribute to healthier gums by keeping the underlying bone strong.

RESEARCH HIGHLIGHT

News alert: National vitamin D deficit. A study from Harvard Medical School found that almost 60% of people admitted to general hospital wards were deficient in vitamin D. Another study from Boston reported that 50% of women with hip fractures were deficient in vitamin D. Drinking milk (or a fortified soy beverage) is the easiest way to meet vitamin D requirements on a daily basis.

Amount of food required for your body to get the same amount of calcium as in one glass of milk

Almonds	**1 cup (250 mL)**
Bok choy	**1 cup (250 mL)**
Broccoli	**2 1/4 cups (550 mL)**
Kale	**1 1/2 cups (375 mL)**
Pinto beans	**4 cups (1 L)**
Spinach	**8 cups (2 L)**
Tofu (made with calcium)	**1/2 cup (125 mL)**

How Much Milk?

The Ultimate Healthy Eating Plan recommends 3 to 4 servings of lower fat milk products each day. (You can consume 2 to 3 servings on the days you have 1 serving of fortified soy milk.)

Your Daily "D"

In order to meet your daily requirement for vitamin D, the Ultimate Healthy Eating Plan recommends that two of your recommended 3 to 4 daily servings be in the form of milk (as opposed to cheese or yogurt) on most days of the week.

Low-fat milk is also lower in calories than most fruit-flavored yogurts or cheese. Fortified soy milk is another way to get vitamin D into your diet.

If you don't drink two glasses of milk (or fortified soy milk) on most days, a multivitamin containing 400 IU of vitamin D is highly recommended. All people over the age of 50 need to consume 2 servings of milk daily, as well as taking a multivitamin since the need for vitamin D increases significantly with age.

But I Can't Drink Milk

True or false: people with lactose intolerance should not consume milk products. False. Several

RESEARCH HIGHLIGHT
When people at high risk for colon cancer increased the intake of low-fat milk products in their diet (1200 mg/day), the precancerous cells in the lining of their colon started acting like healthy cells.

recent, well-controlled studies found that even people who suffer from lactose intolerance (proper term "lactose maldigestion") can consume 1/2 to 1 cup (125 to 250 mL) of milk without symptoms of intolerance as long as they consume it with meals. Solid food slows the digestive process and gives the body more time to digest the lactose. A recent study of African-American girls suffering from lactose maldigestion also found that the colon adapts to milk products when they are consumed on a regular basis. Lastly, most yogurts (those made with bacterial cultures) and hard cheeses (cheddar, Swiss, Colby and Parmesan) contain very little lactose and are well tolerated.

Milk and Prostate Cancer

Do men who drink lots of milk increase their risk of prostate cancer? In the Physicians' Health Study involving more than 21,000 men, those men who consumed more than 600 mg of calcium (more than 2 servings of milk products) daily were 32% more likely to develop prostate cancer. Men who consumed over 2000 mg of calcium daily—from food and supplements combined—were at the highest risk of developing this disease. Researchers speculate that too much calcium in the body slows or even stops the conversion of inactive vitamin D

ONE SERVING OF MILK PRODUCTS	1 cup (250 mL) milk
	1 cup (250 mL) buttermilk
	2 slices (2 oz or 50 g) cheese
	3/4 cup (175 g) yogurt
	4 tbsp (60 mL) grated Parmesan cheese
	1/2 cup (125 mL) ricotta cheese
ONE-HALF SERVING OF MILK PRODUCTS	3/4 cup (175 mL) ice cream
	1/2 cup (125 mL) frozen yogurt
	1 cup (250 mL) cottage cheese

To reduce your intake of saturated fat, choose lower fat milk products. A high intake of saturated fats is associated with an increased risk of heart disease and some cancers. Cheese in particular is a major source of saturated fat in the North American diet.

osteoporosis

QUESTION OF THE DAY

"How come countries like Japan where people don't consume a lot of milk products, have low rates of osteoporosis?" Many factors influence the risk of osteoporosis, including genetics, level of physical activity and vitamin D. And while research shows a lower incidence of hip fractures in Japanese women, some researchers believe the shape of the Asian women's hip (they have a shorter hip axis length) makes their bones less likely to break. It's important to note that Japanese women living in regions where milk intake is higher do have greater bone density. Most important, well-designed clinical studies provide strong evidence of the link between calcium intake and bone health.

YOUR DAILY REQUIREMENT FOR CALCIUM AND VITAMIN D		
Age	Calcium	Vitamin D
1–3	500 mg	5 mcg (200 IU)
4–8	800 mg	5 mcg (200 IU)
9–18	1300 mg	5 mcg (200 IU)
19–50	1000 mg	5 mcg (200 IU)
51–70	1200 mg	10 mcg (400 IU)
71+	1200 mg	15 mcg (600 IU)

One serving of milk products provides about 300 mg of calcium. Most people get about 250 mg of calcium from other foods throughout the day. One serving of milk (not cheese or yogurt) provides about 2.5 mcg (100 IU) of vitamin D.

to its active form. Inside the prostate, the active form of vitamin D is thought to help stop cancer cells from growing and dividing.

Does this mean men should stop drinking milk? The research in this area is preliminary. I believe most men truly benefit from including milk products in their diet. Those with a family history of prostate cancer may choose to limit their consumption to 2 servings daily and meet the rest of their needs through other sources such as fortified soy milk. The most important message here, however, is that taking high-dose calcium supplements may be harmful to men, especially those at high risk for prostate cancer.

Could It Possibly Get Any More Confusing?

Just when you thought nutrition couldn't get any more confusing, it did! Researchers have identified a compound in milk fat called CLA (conjugated linoleic acid). It's also found in beef fat. This compound appears to have many beneficial effects. It may lower your risk of heart disease, boost your immune system, help prevent certain cancers and even help regulate body fat. The downside? Research suggests you have to consume large quantities of high-fat milk products to get enough of it (too many high-fat milk products equals too much saturated fat and calories, which is also linked to a higher risk of disease). Possible solution? Researchers are investigating ways of increasing the amount of CLA in milk products so you can reap the benefits without consuming all that fat. In the meantime, it appears wise to choose

drink more milk

GOOD ADVICE

Do you stop for coffee at your local coffee shop? For more nutrition, including calcium, make your order a café latte. At home, use generous amounts of milk in your coffee or tea.

RESEARCH HIGHLIGHT

The more often you dine away from home, the less likely you are to meet your recommended intake for milk products. Make milk products a part of your life at home and on the road.

GOOD ADVICE

Don't like the taste of milk? Drink chocolate milk (did someone say chocolate?). For fewer calories, make your own (see page 84). Most store-bought, ready-made chocolate milk tends to be a fairly concentrated source of calories.

primarily lower fat milk products. Both skim and 1% milk are considered low in fat. Skim milk contains no CLA, 1% milk contains small amounts. (Can small amounts make a difference? We don't really know.)

Cheese Trivia

Here are some things you should know about cheese:

- Ricotta cheese contains about five times more calcium and three times less salt than cottage cheese.

- Cream cheese is not a good source of calcium. You need to eat about 26 tablespoons (390 mL) of cream cheese to get the same amount of calcium as one glass of milk.

- Most soft cheeses like brie, Camembert, feta and goat's cheese are lower in calcium than hard cheeses like cheddar, Swiss, mozzarella or Parmesan.

- Most processed cheeses, including processed cheese slices, are a source of calcium, but also contain at least twice as much salt.

- If you think most low-fat cheeses taste like rubber (or worse!), choose reduced-fat or "light" cheeses instead. Also consider strong-flavored cheeses like extra sharp cheddar. You tend to be satisfied with less.

The Yogurt Story

When most people think of bacteria they think of something bad or dirty—something to be avoided. And yet more than 500 kinds of bacteria live along your gastrointestinal tract. Many of these bacteria are considered "good" or "friendly." That's because they help you combat the "bad" bacteria that may come your way and also help maintain the health of the cells that line your gastrointestinal tract. While all yogurts are made with active bacterial cultures (yogurt is basically milk fermented by the addition of bacteria), some yogurts also contain added "good" bacteria, referred to as "probiotics." Probiotics are defined as living organisms that can potentially promote health when consumed in sufficient quantity. Bacterial cultures that have been identified as probiotic include Lactobacillus acidophilus, Lactobacillus casei, Lactobacillus rhamnosus GG and Bifidobacterium (try saying these words 10 times fast!). If these bacteria are added to the yogurt their presence is identified on the label or lid of the product. Very preliminary research suggests that consuming probiotics may

RESEARCH HIGHLIGHT
Adults and children who drink more pop drink less milk. What does pop have to offer? About 10 teaspoons (50 mL) of sugar per can and nothing in the way of vitamins and minerals. If you like pop, enjoy it once in a while in moderation. Diet pop is the better choice. Most important: make milk a priority in your diet.

RESEARCH HIGHLIGHT
Attention all parents: if you want your kids to drink milk, drink it yourself.

- help boost the immune system

- reduce intolerance to lactose

- help with diarrhea that results from taking antibiotics (antibiotics kill both good and bad bacteria)

- help with diarrhea caused by an infection or virus

- inhibit certain enzymes that may promote cancer of the colon

- help prevent certain allergies such as eczema (especially if consumed by the mother during pregnancy)

- help increase resistance to immune-related diseases such as inflammatory bowel disease

Many questions still need to be answered, however, and more research is required. How much of these "good" bacteria must be consumed to experience the health benefits? Are certain strains of bacteria more effective than others? Limited data suggest that a daily dose of between 1 billion to 100 billion living micro-organisms may be optimal (it sounds like a lot but remember these bacteria are microscopic in size). Many yogurts from your local supermarket contain less than this.

What's my advice? As the research continues to unfold, we are likely to gain a better understanding of probiotics. We are also more likely to see probiotic yogurts and drinks (containing significant numbers of bacteria) become more widely available, as they currently are in Japan and Europe. In the meantime, when you do consume yogurt, I believe it does make sense to choose brands that contain added probiotic bacteria.

THE ULTIMATE HEALTHY EATING PLAN

Enjoy 3 to 4 servings of lower fat milk products each day. For vitamin D, 2 of those servings should be in the form of milk on most days of the week. One serving of fortified soy milk can be substituted for 1 serving of milk products each day.

SENSATIONAL SOY
AND THE WHOLE
DARN BEAN FAMILY

THE OBJECTIVES OF THE ULTIMATE HEALTHY EATING PLAN ARE TO REDUCE YOUR RISK OF DISEASE BY

optimizing

beans | soy | soy products

MORE BEANS, PLEASE!

Beans, beans, the magical fruit. Dr. George Hosfield, researcher and plant breeder from Michigan State University, states "beans are probably the best human plant food there is." His statement doesn't surprise me. Beans are absolute powerhouses in the nutritional kingdom—loaded with vitamins, minerals and fiber. Beans—especially soybeans—are superstars in the world of disease prevention because of the potent and beneficial plant compounds they contain. Bottom line? There's never bean a better time to make beans a regular part of your diet.

Nutritional All-Stars

Here are beans' nutritional claims to fame:

- Beans contain substantial amounts of the B vitamins—especially folate. Folate (also referred to as folic acid) continues to make headlines in the disease prevention world. It helps prevent serious birth defects during pregnancy, significantly lowers the risk of both heart disease and cancer, and may even help ward off Alzheimer's disease. It's a nutrient most of us simply don't get enough of.

- Beans, especially soybeans, are the best plant source of protein. Protein, among other things, builds skin, muscle, bones and hair. In fact, every cell in our body is constructed from the protein we get from foods.

- Beans contain significant amounts of calcium, iron, copper, zinc, phosphorus, potassium, magnesium and manganese—all essential nutrients for good health. (The absorption of some of

plant-based diet

RESEARCH HIGHLIGHT

Countries such as Japan and China, where people eat lots of soyfoods, have lower rates of breast, uterus, prostate and colon cancer. More than 20 studies, primarily involving Asian people, have found that the consumption of just 1 serving of soy per day is enough to reduce the risk of cancer.

QUESTION OF THE DAY

"Is 'legume' just another word for 'beans'?" When I talk about beans, I'm really referring to the legume family. Legumes, often referred to as dried beans and peas, are edible seeds from the pods of certain plants. The legume family includes peas (such as split peas, chickpeas and black-eyed peas), beans (such as lima, navy, kidney, pinto, black and soybeans) and lentils (such as red, brown and green lentils). Green peas and green beans are considered vegetables.

these nutrients is decreased somewhat because of the presence of certain plant compounds in beans called phytates. However, overall, beans still offer lots of great nutrition.)

- Beans are an excellent source of carbohydrates, the most efficient and preferred source of fuel for our bodies.

- Beans are loaded with fiber. One cup (250 mL) of most beans contains between 9 and 16 grams of fiber. People who eat beans regularly are much more likely to get the recommended 25 to 35 grams of fiber each day. Lots of fiber helps maintain a healthy gastrointestinal tract and helps keep blood cholesterol levels low.

More Beans Please!

The Ultimate Healthy Eating Plan recommends eating beans at least three to five times each week. Beans are considered an alternative to meat. (You need 2 to 3 servings of meat or meat alternatives each day.)

ONE SERVING	1/2 cup (125 mL) beans

Top Six Ways to Say Hello to Beans

1 Bean Dips Such as Hummus (Chickpea Spread)
Bean dips are great with cut-up veggies like carrot sticks or wedges of whole-wheat pita bread. They also make great sandwich fillings. Buy lower fat, ready-made dips or try our delicious Hummus with Roasted Red Peppers (page 229).

2 Roast Them
Here's an amazing recipe! Simply drain and rinse a can (19 oz/540 mL) of chickpeas. Toss with 1 tablespoon (15 mL) extra virgin olive oil and a few shakes of dried rosemary. Add a bit of salt and pepper to taste. Spread on a baking sheet. Bake in a 350°F (180°C) oven for about 45 minutes (longer if you like them really crispy). Let them

RESEARCH HIGHLIGHT
Protein is processed through your kidneys. Plant protein is easier for your kidneys to manage than protein from animals. About one-third of all people with Type I diabetes will eventually develop kidney disease. Researchers believe it would be less likely to develop if these people ate less protein from animal sources and more from plant sources like soy.

QUOTE OF THE DAY
"With the shift towards a more plant-based diet, beans and soy will be potent tools in the treatment and prevention of chronic disease."

Dr. James Anderson, University of Kentucky

RESEARCH HIGHLIGHT
In a study from the United States Department of Agriculture, men followed either a healthy, low-fat diet containing animal protein or a healthy, low-fat diet containing soy protein. Decreases in LDL ("bad") cholesterol levels were significantly greater in those on the soy protein diet.

cool 5 minutes and serve warm. Great for snacking. Kids love them! One 1/2-cup (125-mL) serving contains 170 calories, 5 grams of fiber and 5 grams of fat. Try them today!

3 Super Soup

From minestrone to black bean soup to lentil soup—the options are endless. Research also suggests soup is a super way to fill yourself up with fewer calories. Look for lower sodium options where available.

4 Salads

Toss a handful of canned beans, such as chickpeas or kidney beans, on top of your favorite green salad. For life in the fast lane, ready-made marinated bean salads are a must. Pack them in a small container and enjoy them as part of your brown bag lunch. President's Choice Tex-Mex Bean and Corn Salad is one of my favorites.

5 Chili: Not Just for Super Bowl Parties

Chili is definitely one of the tastiest ways to enjoy beans. The spicier the better! Make a big batch and freeze it for those days when you don't feel like cooking. Try our Out-of-this-World Chili (page 238).

6 Baked Beans

Open a can of baked beans. Put them in a bowl. Heat them in the microwave. Serve with whole-wheat toast, a glass of milk and a piece of fruit. Instant dinner. Kids love them too—especially the after-effects!

Sensational Soy

In the world of beans, there is a super-bean—the soybean. It's nothing short of a super-food when it comes to health. It's wonderful for your heart. It may help you ward off cancer. It may reduce your risk of osteoporosis and more. What makes the soybean such an all-star when it comes to disease prevention? Most of the disease-fighting benefits appear to come from estrogen-like plant compounds called isoflavones, which are found in high quantities in soy protein.

Soy Healthy for Your Heart

Soy helps reduce your risk of heart disease by

- decreasing LDL ("bad") cholesterol levels

- preventing damage to LDL cholesterol (when LDL gets damaged or "oxidized" it is more likely to cause plaque to build up on artery walls)

- reducing triglycerides in your blood

eat beans

GOOD ADVICE

Eat beans. Manage your waistline. High-fiber foods such as beans deliver more bulk with fewer calories. They take longer to digest and leave you feeling more satisfied (you feel full for a longer period of time). They may also influence appetite by altering certain hormones, and they contain protein (a bit of protein with each meal helps keep hunger at bay).

GOOD ADVICE

Canned beans are a nutritious and time-saving alternative to cooking beans from scratch. The downside? They're loaded with salt. Most canned beans contain about 400 mg of sodium per 1/2 cup (125 mL) serving. By draining the canning liquid and rinsing, however, you'll cut the salt by almost half.

RESEARCH HIGHLIGHT

Prevent and manage diabetes with beans. Beans take longer to digest than many other foods and have a low glycemic index (they don't cause a rapid increase in blood sugar). Soybeans, in particular, have been shown to improve sensitivity to insulin (less insulin is required to maintain a healthy blood sugar level).

- helping prevent blood clots from forming

- keeping blood vessels healthy and dilated

While higher levels of soy are required for significant decreases in blood cholesterol (25 grams of soy protein per day or about 3 servings of soy), a daily serving of soy is still beneficial for the heart.

The Cancer Connection

Recent studies suggest that soy may reduce the risk of hormone-sensitive cancers. In studies involving human and animal cells, the isoflavone genistein consistently kills breast and prostate cancer cells. When animals are fed a high soy diet and injected with cancer-causing substances, tumors take much longer to develop and are much smaller in size. One of the ways that genistein is thought to work is by inhibiting certain enzymes involved in the production of hormones. High blood levels of estrogen, for example, are thought to stimulate the growth and spread of tumor cells. Preliminary research also suggests that for full breast cancer protection, girls should eat soy prior to puberty (when breast tissue is still forming). In other words, a daily serving of soy appears to be beneficial for both children and adults.

How Much Soy?

The Ultimate Healthy Eating Plan recommends 1 to 2 servings of soy each day.

ONE SERVING OF SOY	1 cup (250 mL) soy milk (fortified with calcium, vitamin D, vitamin B12)
	1/2 cup (125 mL) tofu
	3 tbsp (45 mL) soy nuts
	1 veggie burger (or other meat replacement product made with soy protein—look for those containing about 10 grams of soy protein/serving)

For the more advanced soy enthusiast (with access to lots of good soy recipes), each of the following equals one serving of soy:

ONE SERVING OF SOY	1/2 cup (125 mL) soybeans (green or mature)
	1/2 cup (125 mL) cooked textured vegetable protein
	1/2 cup (125 mL) tempeh
	1/4 cup (50 mL) soy flour
	3 tbsp (45 mL) miso

isoflavones

RESEARCH HIGHLIGHT
Reduce your risk of osteoporosis. A study involving almost 500 postmenopausal Japanese women found that women who consumed the highest levels of isoflavones from soyfoods had significantly thicker bones than women who consumed the lowest levels. Isoflavones appear to stimulate bone formation, as well as help reduce bone loss.

QUESTION OF THE DAY
"If I eat soy, can I reduce menopause-related symptoms like hot flashes?" The isoflavones in soy (also called phyto-estrogens) are similar in structure to the hormone estrogen. Although some studies support the use of soy in reducing the number and severity of hot flashes, other studies do not.

What we do know is that in Japan, where soy is a regular part of the diet, there is no word in their vocabulary for hot flashes.

Fortified soy milk can be used as a replacement to cow's milk (although, for most people, I still recommend some dairy in the diet). Other soy products should be considered a replacement to meat.

Why 1–2 Soy Servings?

Asian countries that enjoy soy as a regular part of their diet, such as Japan, have lower rates of disease. Most Asian populations consume between 20 and 40 mg of isoflavones daily, which translates into about 1 to 2 servings of soy (or about 10 to 20 grams of soy protein). While some studies suggest higher intakes may be helpful for full protection from disease, further research is required before recommendations can be made. For most people, focusing on eating a wide variety of healthy foods—as opposed to a single food item like soy—makes the most sense for good health.

Soy Tasty

Do you love the health benefits of soy but not the taste? If so, you're not alone. Often people complain they find soy a less-than-tasty addition to their diet. It doesn't have to be that way. Here are six fast, easy and tasty ways to enjoy soy:

1 Go Nuts

Roasted soy nuts are tasty, easy and portable. They taste sort of like peanuts, but crunchier. They're widely available in supermarkets, and some stores sell seasoned varieties, like honey-roasted or barbecue flavor. They're great for on-the-run snack attacks: keep a stash in your bag, briefcase or glove compartment of your car. You can also toss them into salads, cooked veggie dishes or stir-fries.

2 Did You Say Chocolate?

If you don't like the taste of regular or vanilla soy milk, how about strawberry or chocolate flavored (my favorite, of course). I enjoy chocolate soy milk heated in the microwave just before bedtime—a few mini-marshmallows on top are always an option. If you're used to the taste of cow's milk, start with a half soy milk, half cow's milk combo. Coffee-lovers can also heat 1 cup (250 mL) of plain or vanilla soy milk in the microwave and stir in a teaspoon (5 mL) of instant coffee (add coffee to chocolate soy milk for a mocha soy latte). Ready-made, coffee-flavored soy milks are also available.

3 Have a Smoothie

Smoothies get top scores for taste and popularity. You must (and I mean must!) try the Super Chocolate Banana Soy Shake (page 245) and the Super Soy Strawberry Smoothie (page 247). So good!

soy protein

GOOD ADVICE

The beneficial plant compounds found in soy protein—isoflavones—are now widely available in pill form. These supplements are not recommended. Eating whole foods that contain soy protein is recommended. Not only does the protein in soy appear to enhance the action of isoflavones, researchers believe soy protein may contain other compounds that also reduce the risk of disease. The safety of high-dose isoflavone supplements is also unknown.

QUESTION OF THE DAY

"Is it safe to eat soy that has been genetically modified?" Overall, I believe genetically modified foods are safe. Biotechnology also helps increase food production, reduce the use of pesticides and benefits farmers and the environment.

4 Pudding Please

Although a chocolate lover at heart, I love butterscotch pudding made with soy milk. Buy powdered pudding mixes and use plain or vanilla soy milk instead of cow's milk. For best results, use the type of pudding mix you heat on the stove. A half cup (125 mL) of pudding equals 1/2 serving of soy. You can also substitute soy milk for cow's milk in other recipes like pancakes or french toast.

5 The Joy of Soy

There are plenty of processed soy products out there, and they're available in most supermarkets. Yves, a Vancouver-based company, sells everything from burgers to lasagna to ground-meat replacements (www.yves.veggie.com). Another Canadian company, SoSoya+ also makes a variety of products including SoSoya+ Slices. They're great for using in stir-fries instead of meat (for more information, visit www.sosoyaplus.com). Because the protein and isoflavone content of these products varies widely, look for those that list soy flour, soy protein isolate or textured soy protein as the first or second ingredient.

6 Green Soybeans

These delicious soybeans, also referred to as edamamé, are harvested when the beans are still green and sweet tasting. If you can't find them

ISOFLAVONE CONTENT OF DIFFERENT SOY FOODS

3 tbsp (45 mL) soy nuts	41 mg
1/4 cup (50 mL) soy flour	33 mg
1/2 cup (125 mL) uncooked tofu	29 mg
1/2 cup (125 mL) uncooked tempeh	36 mg
1 cup (250 mL) soy milk	24 mg
3 tbsp (45 mL) miso	22 mg
1 veggie burger (90 g)	8 mg

Source: USDA Isoflavone Database

Note: Most Asian populations consume between 20 and 40 mg of isoflavones daily. The isoflavone content varies widely among different soybean varieties and from product to product based on the manufacturing process and source of soy protein. Soy sauce and soybean oil are not a source of isoflavones.

soybeans & soy milk

QUESTION OF THE DAY

"Are soybeans high in fat?" Generally, beans are low in fat. There is, however, one exception: the soybean. Over 40% of the calories in soybeans come from fat. The good news is that soy is low in saturated fat, the not-so-healthy fat found in higher fat meat and dairy products. To limit calories, however, it is still a good idea to choose lower fat versions of soy products, like low-fat tofu and soy milk, more often. Limit higher fat soy products like roasted soy nuts to 1 serving per day.

RESEARCH HIGHLIGHT

In the Seventh Day Adventist Study involving over 12,000 men, those who drank soy milk more than once a day had a 70% lower risk of prostate cancer.

fresh, you can can find them frozen in most supermarkets. Boil them as directed. Add them to stir-fries, pastas, salads or chill them and serve as a snack.

The Gas You Pass

Fact: beans give you gas (technical term: flatulence). If it's a problem for you, there are two options. Option one: try Beano, a product available at most supermarkets and drugstores. It contains the enzyme that helps break down the hard-to-digest sugars in beans that cause gas. It works! Option two: enjoy beans with those who know and love you best.

QUESTION OF THE DAY

"Is it true that people with a family history of breast cancer should not eat soy?" This is a difficult question to answer based on the research currently available. Soy has generally been linked to lower rates of breast cancer, especially when consumed over a lifetime. In a few studies, however, isoflavone supplements have been found to stimulate the growth of breast cancer cells. For this reason, soy researchers generally suggest that women at a high risk for breast cancer, women who are taking the drug tamoxifen, and women who have (or have had) hormone-dependent breast cancer may want to limit themselves to no more than a few servings of soy a week. Most important, women with a history of breast cancer should avoid taking soy supplements; many contain isoflavones far in excess of the amounts possible to get through diet.

FANTASTIC FISH

THE OBJECTIVES OF THE ULTIMATE HEALTHY EATING PLAN ARE TO REDUCE YOUR RISK OF DISEASE BY

optimizing

omega-3 fats found in higher fat fish

AN INCREDIBLE FAT

There is one overwhelming reason to eat fish, specifically higher fat fish such as salmon, mackerel, herring and rainbow trout. It's the fat. The fat in fish, referred to as the omega-3 fats, are spectacular (bet you never thought you'd hear that word used to describe fat!). They've earned all-star status on the disease-protection checklist. Their greatest claim to fame is their ability to protect your heart. Beyond that, they may reduce your risk of some cancers, inflammatory disorders such as arthritis, and macular degeneration—the leading cause of blindness in older adults. They may also reduce your risk of depression as well as age-related declines in your mental functioning, including Alzheimer's disease.

Outstanding Protection for Your Heart

Your heart loves the omega-3 fats found in fish. People who eat fish regularly (higher fat fish, that is!) are less likely to have a heart attack or a stroke. If a heart attack does occur, they reduce their risk of dying from it by as much as 50% or more. In addition, damage to the heart muscle is greatly reduced. How does fish protect your heart? In a number of ways. When you eat higher fat fish you

- decrease the stickiness of your blood (this means that blood clots, often the first step in a heart attack, are less likely to form)

- help your heart keep a strong and regular beat (irregular heart beats are another leading cause of heart attacks)

- keep your artery walls relaxed and dilated

- lower the level of triglycerides in your blood—another type of blood fat linked to heart disease

omega-3 fats

QUOTE OF THE DAY
"Omega-3 fats have immense public health significance for the control of the current epidemic of heart disease."

William Connor, *American Journal of Clinical Nutrition*, October 2001

RESEARCH HIGHLIGHT
An Australian study involving almost 600 children found that children who regularly consumed higher fat fish had a four times lower risk of developing asthma. Omega-3 fats in fish may prevent the development of asthma by reducing airway inflammation and responsiveness. Moral of the story? Eat fish, breathe easy.

RESEARCH HIGHLIGHT
Doctors at two Copenhagen hospitals confirmed that eating fish regularly helps prevent narrowing of the arteries due to the buildup of plaque (fatty deposits). The doctors performed 40 autopsies and determined that the degree of plaque present in the coronary arteries was inversely proportional to the amount of omega-3 fat from fish in the fatty tissue.

- reduce inflammation of the artery wall, which in turn reduces the buildup of plaque or fatty deposits (many researchers now believe that inflammation plays a key role in the development of heart disease)

Fight Cancer with Omega-3s

Evidence suggests that the diet of early humans—and which our genetic makeup was programmed for—contained equal amounts of omega-3 fats and omega-6 fats. Today, it appears many people may be consuming significantly more of the omega-6 fats (found in safflower oil, sunflower oil, corn oil and many products made with these oils) and less of the omega-3 fats. Research suggests that the omega-3 fats (especially when balanced with the omega-6 fats) may play an important role in reducing the risk of some cancers—especially cancers of the breast, colon and possibly the prostate. They appear to work by inhibiting certain compounds involved in the development and spread of cancerous tumors. Further research will tell us more.

Arthritis and More

The omega-3 fats in fish reduce inflammation. Inflammation is your body's response to the injury of body tissues. It often involves pain and swelling. It is associated with diseases such as arthritis, Crohn's disease, ulcerative colitis, nephropathy, psoriasis, asthma and even heart disease. Eating fish regularly may help in the management of these diseases. In some cases, fish oil supplements may be beneficial. For example, research suggests that a daily dose of about 3 grams of fish oil may be optimal for reducing the pain and stiffness associated with rheumatoid arthritis (the benefits of which are usually not seen until after about 12 weeks). People who suffer from heart disease, especially those who have survived a heart attack, may want to consider taking 1 gram of fish oil daily. People who take fish oil supplements may

QUESTION OF THE DAY

"I don't like fish. Can I get my omega-3 fats from foods like flax, walnuts and canola oil instead?" In the optimal disease-prevention plan, both fish source and plant source omega-3 fats are included. Plant-source omega-3 fats appear to be most important for helping your heart keep a strong and regular beat. (They can also be converted to fish-type omega-3 fats in your body, but only to a limited degree). Fish-source omega-3 fats (also referred to as EPA/DHA) are incorporated directly into various cell membranes throughout your body and, as such, appear to play a much wider role in the prevention of disease. Suggestion: eat your flax, walnuts and canola oil, but be sure to also enjoy some of the outstanding fish recipes in this book. (Salmon is one of the richest and possibly most delicious ways to get your omega-3 fats.) We'll make a fish-lover out of you yet!

also need to take a supplement of about 200 IU of vitamin E (fish oil supplements appear to lower blood levels of vitamin E). Further research will help clarify our understanding of these diseases and the role that fish and fish oils have to play.

For most people, the best advice is to eat fish, not take fish oil supplements. Fish is an important source of other nutrients such as protein, vitamin B12, vitamin B6, niacin, phosphorus, magnesium, selenium and iron. Have some fish today!

Protect Your Eyes

The omega-3 fats in fish are vital components of various cell membranes throughout your body. They are particularly abundant in the retina of your eye. Research suggests that those who eat fish regularly are less likely to develop age-related macular degeneration. This disease is the leading cause of blindness in older adults. It is characterized by fuzziness, shadows or other distortions in the center of vision. Perhaps seafood should be called see-food (chuckle, chuckle).

Brain Food

The omega-3 fats in fish are incorporated into various cell membranes in your brain. Preliminary research from the Rotterdam Study and the Zutphen Elderly Study suggests that those who eat fish regularly are less likely to suffer from a decline in age-related thinking skills such as memory. The risk of developing Alzheimer's disease also appears to be lower. Lastly, several studies have linked low intakes of omega-3 fats to higher rates of depression. Moral of the story: eat fish, think clearly, be happy!

Just Twice a Week!

The Ultimate Healthy Eating Plan recommends eating 2 servings of higher fat fish each week.

ONE SERVING OF HIGHER FAT FISH	3 oz (85 g) fish (about the size of a deck of cards)
	3/4 cup (175 mL) flaked or canned fish

Higher fat fish include salmon, herring, mackerel, rainbow trout and bluefin tuna. Anchovies and pickled herring are also high in omega-3 fats; however, they are very high in salt. Enjoy them on occasion.

Top Eight Seafood Eating Tips

1 Most frozen fish sticks and fast-food fish sandwiches are a poor source of omega-3 fats. The type of fish used is not high in fat, and some of

heart disease

RESEARCH HIGHLIGHT
In the Physician's Health Study, men who ate fish once or more each week were 52% less likely to die of a heart attack compared to men who ate fish once a month or less.

RESEARCH HIGHLIGHT
In the Seven Countries Study, eating higher fat fish was linked to a lower risk of dying from heart disease. No association was found between eating lean fish and heart disease. Moral of the story: while lean fish is still a very healthy choice, for optimal protection from disease, be sure to enjoy higher fat fish on a regular basis.

RESEARCH HIGHLIGHT
In a recent study involving two African villages, the risk of heart disease was lower in a fish-eating village as compared to a vegetarian village.

the omega-3 fats are lost during processing (not to mention that most of these products are loaded with nasty, not-good-for-your-heart hydrogenated fats).

2 Most of the fresh tuna on restaurant menus and at fish counters is yellowfin tuna, which is not high in omega-3 fats. A much better choice is bluefin tuna, which is served at some upscale restaurants. When choosing canned tuna, pick albacore tuna (labeled "white" or "white albacore" tuna). It contains more omega-3 fats than other types.

3 If you don't want dry, tough fish, don't over-cook it! Most fish requires just 10 minutes of cooking time for each inch (2.5 cm) of thickness. Properly cooked fish will flake easily with a fork.

4 Frozen fish (not breaded) is a tasty and conven-ient alternative to fresh fish. I always have frozen salmon fillets in my freezer for quick and easy dinners.

5 It's okay to enjoy shrimp! Yes, they contain cho-lesterol, but they are very low in fat and calories. While cholesterol should be consumed in mod-eration, it's the saturated fats (found in higher fat milk and meat products) and hydrogenated

GOOD ADVICE

Pregnant and nursing women—eat your fish. The omega-3 fats in fish are essential for the healthy development of your baby's brain and eyes. This development takes place in the womb and throughout the first year of your baby's life. But avoid shark, swordfish, king mackerel and tilefish; they may contain unsafe amounts of mercury. Tuna may also contain mercury, but in smaller amounts. Eat tuna no more than once a week.

RESEARCH HIGHLIGHT

An Australian study involving more than 3500 older adults found that eating fish just one to three times per month appeared to protect against age-related macular degeneration, the leading cause of blindness in older adults.

no fish tale

RESEARCH HIGHLIGHT

In a study involving more than 6000 men from Sweden, those men who regularly ate higher fat fish (about 2 to 3 servings per week), reduced their risk of prostate cancer by 50%.

GOOD ADVICE

Do you suffer from diabetes? If so, eat your fish! People with diabetes are much more likely to develop heart disease. Fish is the all-star protector of the heart.

RESEARCH HIGHLIGHT

In the Nurses' Health Study, women who ate fish two to four times per week had an almost 30% lower risk of stroke than those who ate fish less than once a month.

fats (found in deep-fried fast food, hard margarine and many processed foods) that are most harmful to health.

6   All shellfish, including shrimp, crab, clams, oysters, lobster, mussels and scallops, are low in fat and rich in protein, iron, copper and zinc. Enjoy.

7   Eating raw seafood like sushi is risky. There's always a chance you might get sick. Even the freshest fish may contain bacteria, parasites and other potentially harmful organisms. While it's true that well-trained sushi chefs know how to purchase and handle fish so as to minimize the risk, there is still no guarantee of safety. Raw clams, oysters and mussels are particularly dangerous.

8   Check with the health department in your area before you eat fish caught in local streams and lakes. They may contain pollutants that are harmful to health. Generally, the fish you purchase at most supermarkets can be considered safe.

THE ULTIMATE HEALTHY EATING PLAN

Enjoy 2 servings of higher fat fish like salmon, mackerel, herring or rainbow trout each week.

RESEARCH HIGHLIGHT
A recent study compared the annual incidence of major depression in nine countries with the consumption of fish. Results: a high incidence of depression was found in countries where people ate less fish. Japan, which has one of the leading fish-eating populations in the world, had the lowest incidence of major depression. While various factors can impact depression, more and more research suggests a link between omega-3 fats and your mood.

QUESTION OF THE DAY
"Is smoked salmon a good source of omega-3 fats?" Unfortunately, no. Smoked salmon contains less than one-quarter of the omega-3 fats found in fresh salmon. Much of the beneficial fats are lost during the smoking process.

OMEGA-3 CONTENT OF SEAFOOD (PER 3-OZ/85-G PORTION)

High Source		Low Source	
Salmon, Atlantic	1.8 g	Flatfish (flounder/sole)	0.4 g
Anchovy, canned in oil, drained	1.7 g	Crab, Alaska king	0.4 g
Herring, Atlantic	1.7 g	Halibut, Atlantic and Pacific	0.4 g
Mackerel, Pacific and jack	1.6 g	Oysters	0.4 g
Salmon, Chinook	1.5 g	Sea trout	0.4 g
Salmon, pink, canned	1.4 g	Smoked salmon	0.4 g
Herring, Atlantic, pickled	1.2 g	Whiting	0.4 g
Tuna, bluefin	1.2 g	Scallops	0.3 g
Salmon, coho	1.1 g	Shrimp	0.3 g
Salmon, sockeye, canned	1.0 g	Snapper	0.3 g
Trout, rainbow	1.0 g	Perch	0.3 g
Mackerel, Atlantic	1.0 g	Catfish	0.2 g
		Fish sticks	0.2 g
		Grouper	0.2 g
		Haddock	0.2 g
Moderate Source		Tuna, light, canned in water	0.2 g
Bluefish	0.9 g	Tuna, yellowfin	0.2 g
Sardines canned in oil, drained	0.8 g	Cod, Atlantic	0.1 g
Smelt, rainbow	0.8 g	Lobster	0.1 g
Tuna, white, canned in water, drained	0.7 g	Mahi mahi	0.1 g
Bass, freshwater	0.7 g	Pike, northern	0.1 g
Sea bass	0.7 g	Orange roughy	0.0 g
Swordfish	0.7 g		
Mussels	0.7 g		
Pollock, Atlantic	0.5 g		

Source: USDA Nutrient Database

THE **MEAT, POULTRY** AND **EGG** STORY

THE OBJECTIVES OF THE ULTIMATE HEALTHY EATING PLAN ARE TO REDUCE YOUR RISK OF DISEASE BY

moderating

lean meat | poultry | eggs

WHERE'S THE BEEF?

Let's start with the meat story. Does meat (beef, pork, poultry) fit into an eating plan focused on reducing your risk of disease? Here are three thought-provoking facts to consider:

1 Vegetarians are significantly less likely to suffer from heart disease than meat-eaters.

2 Meat-eaters—especially red-meat-eaters—are more likely to develop cancer of the colon. They may also be at higher risk for cancers of the breast, stomach and prostate. (How you cook your meat appears to influence this risk.)

3 Ground beef and processed meats (luncheon meats, bacon, sausages, hot dogs) are major sources of saturated fat in the typical North American diet. For optimal protection from disease, we should limit our intake of saturated fat.

Before you conclude there is no place for meat in a diet focused on health, also consider the following five facts:

1 Evidence suggests that the diet upon which humans evolved included meat. The meat consumed was primarily wild game, which is extremely lean.

GOOD ADVICE
One of the top sources of saturated fat (the not-so-healthy-for-your-heart fat) in the typical North American diet is ground beef. When you do buy ground beef, always buy extra lean. Be sure to brown the meat and drain off the fat before adding it to foods like chili, spaghetti sauce or shepherd's pie. And try some of the meatless recipes in this book. Our Out-of-this-World Chili (page 238), made with beans and a soy meat-replacement is out-of-this-world delicious!

2 People in countries like Japan and those of the Mediterranean, which are known for their low rates of disease, eat meat. Generally, however, they eat significantly less meat than do people in many countries with higher rates of disease. Japan, for example, has traditionally consumed about one-third as much meat as the United States.

3 Meat, especially beef, provides substantial amounts of highly available (easily absorbed) iron and zinc compared to other sources. Many people—especially children, teenaged girls and women of childbearing age—are at risk for iron and zinc deficiencies. Even mild deficiencies are linked to poor growth, impaired learning ability, reduced work performance and lower resistance to infections.

4 Meat is an important source of vitamin B12 in our diets. A significant number of people—especially older adults—do not get enough vitamin B12 in their diets.

5 Research supports that lean meat can fit into a heart-healthy diet—especially when that diet is also rich in health-protective foods like whole grains, beans, vegetables and fruit.

Bottom line: small quantities of lean meat can fit in a healthy diet.

Be a Lean Meat Eater
The Ultimate Healthy Eating Plan recommends eating lean meat and poultry.

Generally, loin and round cuts of beef or pork are the leanest. Sirloin, sirloin tip and tenderloin are all good examples of lower fat loin cuts. Inside round, eye of round and outside round are good examples of lower fat round cuts. For chicken or turkey, breast meat is the leanest. However, all cuts can be enjoyed as long as the skin is removed. About 50% to 80% of the fat is in the skin and it's the not-so-healthy-for-your-heart, saturated kind! Choose low-fat luncheon meats such as lean roast beef, turkey, chicken and ham (choose lower sodium brands where available). Extra lean ground meat or poultry is also acceptable (just don't forget to brown and drain the meat).

Attention All Barbecue Lovers
How often do you barbecue? Do you marinate your meat before you grill it? Do you like your meat well done? Your answers to these questions and others may influence your risk of cancer—

RESEARCH HIGHLIGHT
In the Seven Countries Study, death from heart disease was found to vary greatly in different countries, ranging from 27% of the population in east Finland to 3% in the island of Crete (Greece). Higher intakes of animal foods (excluding fish) were linked to higher rates of heart disease. Higher intakes of plant foods (vegetables, fruit, beans, grains) were linked to lower rates of heart disease.

QUOTE OF THE DAY
"A meal that's both tasty and cancer protective should contain a high proportion of foods like fruits, vegetables and grains that are rich in cancer-fighting substances and a much smaller proportion of meat."

Dr. Ritva Butrum, American Institute for Cancer Research

RESEARCH HIGHLIGHT
A review of 45 studies supports the hypothesis that meat consumption is associated with a modest increase in colon cancer risk. This association, however, seems to have been found more consistently for red meat and processed meats.

particularly cancers of the colon, breast, stomach and prostate. When meat (red meat, poultry or fish) is cooked at high temperatures, as it is during barbecuing, broiling or frying, cancer-causing compounds called "heterocyclic amines" (HCAs) are formed. When the fat from meat, poultry or fish drips onto hot coals, another type of cancer-causing compound called polycyclic aromatic hydrocarbons (PAHs) are formed. These compounds are deposited onto the food when the smoke rises. The good news is you can reduce the formation of these compounds by following a few simple rules.

Cooking Tips for Healthy Meat Eating (When Grilling, Broiling or Frying)

1 Marinate your meat before you cook it. This significantly reduces the formation of cancer-causing compounds. Herbs, spices, oils and acidic ingredients (like vinegar and citrus juices) all seem to contribute to the prevention of cancer-causing compounds.

2 Trim the fat. Choose lean, well-trimmed meats to grill. They have less fat to drip onto the flames. Remove the skin from poultry.

3 For faster cooking times, keep meat portions small. Skewered kebobs cook the fastest on the grill. Stir-frying small strips of meat is your best option when frying.

4 Consider precooking meats in the oven or microwave. Grill them briefly for flavor.

5 Keep flipping. Research suggests that cooking hamburger patties at a lower temperature and turning them often accelerates the cooking process and helps prevent the formation of cancer-causing compounds. Be sure to cook them until the centers are no longer pink and the juices show no pink color. This ensures that any bacteria present are killed. Steaks can still be enjoyed rare or medium as any bacteria present is only on the surface.

6 Remove all charred or burned portions of food before eating.

7 Braising, stewing and roasting (baking) meat are considered safer cooking methods for meat.

8 Don't worry about grilling your veggies or fruit. Only meat, fish and poultry form cancer-causing compounds during cooking.

RESEARCH HIGHLIGHT
In the Nurses' Health Study involving almost 80,000 women, those who ate more red meat and less chicken and fish were at significantly greater risk of colon cancer. While there is strong support for including fish in a disease-prevention diet, research also suggests that choosing lean poultry more often than red meat also makes sense.

RESEARCH HIGHLIGHT
In a U.S. study involving more than 900 women, those who said they ate lots of charred and grilled meats were twice as likely to get breast cancer as women who rarely or never did.

Meat: How Much? How Often?

The Ultimate Healthy Eating Plan recommends eating no more than 1 serving of lean meat each day. When you do eat meat, choose chicken or turkey (skin removed) more often. Limit your intake of red meat to no more than twice a week. Enjoy meatless days at least once a week. Have beans, fish or nuts instead.

ONE SERVING OF MEAT	2 to 3 oz (60 to 85 g) lean meat or poultry (3 oz/85 g of meat is about the size of a deck of cards) 2 slices lean cold cuts (3 in x 3 in x 1/4 in/7 1/2 cm x 7 1/2 cm x 1/2 cm)

Have Eggs Instead?

The Ultimate Healthy Eating Plan recommends eating eggs no more than three to four times a week.

ONE SERVING	One egg. Always choose omega-3 eggs.

Let's talk eggs—the good and the maybe-not-so-good. Here are the facts:

1 Eggs are nutrient dense. They contain more than 15 nutrients that are important to good health all in one neat, little package (all for only 70 calories). With the exception of protein, most of the nutrients are found in the yolk.

2 Eggs are a good source of the carotenoids lutein and zeaxanthin—compounds that are also found in dark leafy greens and linked to a reduced risk of age-related macular degeneration, a leading cause of blindness in older adults.

3 Eggs are rich in choline—a nutrient required for the normal function of all cells. Research suggests that choline may be particularly important for early brain development. Pregnant women should therefore eat eggs.

4 Eggs are easy on the pocketbook and make for fast, easy meals.

5 Eggs contain cholesterol. The health risks of foods that are rich in cholesterol is an ongoing topic of debate among researchers. While research suggests that most people can safely consume eggs in moderation (even one egg per day), some people are more sensitive than others to the cholesterol in food. These people—called cholesterol-responders—experience a very

if you're a vegetarian

RESEARCH HIGHLIGHT

A review of five studies involving more than 76,000 men and women found that vegetarians were 24% less likely to die from heart disease compared to nonvegetarians with similar lifestyles. Vegetarians who also ate fish (pesco-vegetarians) or who ate milk and eggs (lacto-ovo vegetarians) were 34% less likely to die from heart disease. If you're considering a vegetarian lifestyle, be sure to replace the meat in your diet with beans (including soy or tofu), nuts (including peanut butter) and seeds. Eggs and fish are also replacements to meat.

significant increase in blood cholesterol levels when they regularly eat cholesterol-rich foods like eggs. People with diabetes—especially if they are overweight—appear to be more likely to fall into this category.

6 One of the best reasons to limit the eggs in your diet is to make more room for health-protective foods like fish, nuts and beans (these foods are all considered alternatives to meat).

7 Chickens fed a diet rich in flaxseed produce eggs that are 8 to 10 times higher in beneficial omega-3 fats (these fats are discussed in detail in the Fantastic Fish chapter) than regular eggs. These omega-3 eggs are a healthier choice than regular eggs. They usually contain significantly more vitamin E as well. It is still important, however to get omega-3 fats from other foods like fish, flax and canola oil in order to optimize your intake.

THE ULTIMATE HEALTHY EATING PLAN

Enjoy no more than 1 serving of lean meat or poultry (with the skin removed) each day. Choose chicken or turkey more often. Limit your intake of red meat to no more than twice a week. Enjoy eggs no more than three to four times a week and always choose omega-3 eggs. Enjoy meatless days regularly. Have beans, fish or nuts instead.

eggs and cholesterol

RESEARCH HIGHLIGHT
Based on the Nurses' Health Study and the Health Professionals Follow-Up Study involving over 115,000 women and men, no evidence was found of a significant overall link between egg consumption and the risk of heart disease or stroke. Higher egg consumption was linked to a higher risk of heart disease in people with diabetes.

RESEARCH HIGHLIGHT
In a large review of 224 studies covering more than 30 years of research, it was demonstrated that dietary cholesterol (the cholesterol found in food) has only a limited effect on blood cholesterol (the amount of cholesterol in your blood). Saturated fats (found in higher fat meat and dairy products) and hydrogenated fats (found in deep-fried fast foods, hard margarine and many processed foods) are much more likely to cause an increase in blood cholesterol levels. Foods like beans, whole grains, vegetables and fruit can all help lower blood cholesterol levels.

GO **NUTS**!

THE OBJECTIVES OF THE ULTIMATE HEALTHY EATING PLAN ARE TO REDUCE YOUR RISK OF DISEASE BY

optimizing

nuts

NUTS: HEROES NOT VILLAINS

Perhaps one of the most unexpected findings in nutrition research in the past decade is that nuts are good for you—really good for you! Perhaps even more exciting is that most people (me included!) love them. Nuts' most deserving reputation comes from their ability to protect your heart. Five large studies (Adventist Health Study, Iowa Women's Health Study, Nurses' Health Study, Physician's Health Study, CARE study) have reported that regular nut eaters have significantly lower rates of heart disease. The relationship between nuts and heart health is remarkably strong and consistent. People who eat nuts regularly are much less likely to have a heart attack and much less likely to die of one. Nut-eaters, not surprisingly, also appear to live longer. Go nuts!

Heart-Healthy

How do nuts protect your heart? Similar to other health-protective foods, nuts contain a very complex mix of nutrients and plant compounds—all of which appear to play a role in optimal health. Nuts are generally rich in

- monounsaturated fats, similar to those found in olive and canola oil (these fats help lower total and LDL, or "bad", cholesterol levels)

- vitamin E, a powerful antioxidant that appears to help protect arterial walls from damage

- folate (folic acid), which lowers blood levels of homocysteine (believed to damage blood vessel walls and encourage the buildup of plaque on artery walls)

- arginine, a building block of protein and precursor to nitric oxide, a potent dilator of blood vessel walls

RESEARCH HIGHLIGHT
In the Adventist Health Study involving over 31,000 men and women, researchers looked at 65 different food items to see which foods were most beneficial for heart health. Nuts came out at the top of the list. People who consumed nuts five or more times a week reduced their risk of heart disease by about 50% compared to those who ate nuts less than once a week. Those who ate nuts one to four times a week reduced their risk by about 25%.

RESEARCH HIGHLIGHT
In the Iowa Women's Health Study involving almost 35,000 postmenopausal women, those who consumed nuts and seeds more than once per week experienced a 40% reduction in heart disease risk compared to those who ate nuts less frequently. There was no significant health benefit to those who consumed nuts only a few times per month.

RESEARCH HIGHLIGHT
Preliminary research suggests that plant compounds in nuts may help reduce the risk of cancers such as colon, prostate and breast cancer. Further research will tell us more.

- fiber, including soluble fiber, which helps lower blood cholesterol

- nutrients such as copper, magnesium, potassium, selenium, all of which play important roles in heart health

- plant compounds such as flavonoids and sterols, which may help lower blood cholesterol and reduce the formation of blood clots

The Nut Plan

The Ultimate Healthy Eating Plan recommends eating 1/2 to 1 serving of nuts five times per week. Consider them as an alternative to meat. Eat only small quantities.

Do not consume more than 1 serving per day (most women and anyone watching their weight should consume only 1/2 serving)—the fat and calories add up quickly. For example, while one handful of most nuts is about 175 calories and 16 grams of fat, three to four handfuls gets you closer to 700 calories and over 60 grams of fat. Moral of the story: don't sit next to the nut bowl.

Good, Better, Best . . .

Are some nuts healthier than other nuts? Here are the nut facts:

| ONE SERVING OF NUTS | 1 oz (30 g) nuts—a small handful or about 1/4 cup (50 mL) |
| | 2 tbsp (25 mL) peanut butter—about the size of a ping-pong ball |

To be even more specific,

ONE SERVING OF NUTS IS ABOUT	6–8	Brazil nuts
	10–12	macadamia nuts
	14	walnut halves
	18	cashews
	20	pecan halves
	20	hazelnuts
	24	almonds
	32	peanuts
	47	pistachio nuts
	160	pine nuts

- Overall, most nuts contain a nutful of good nutrition including nutrients like protein, manganese, copper, magnesium, phosphorus, zinc, vitamin E, selenium, folate, boron, thiamin and niacin.

- Most seeds, especially sunflower seeds, tend to be higher in the omega-6 fats. We want to moderate our intake of omega-6 fats and get more

GOOD ADVICE
Coconuts should not be on your eat-more-often list. Almost 90% of the fats they contain are the unhealthy-for-your-heart, saturated kind.

RESEARCH HIGHLIGHT
In a follow-up to the Adventist Health Study, involving men and women 84 years of age and older, eating nuts five or more times per week decreased the risk of death from heart disease by almost 40% compared to those who consumed nuts less than once a week. Moral of the story: it's never too late to go nuts!

RESEARCH HIGHLIGHT
In yet another follow-up to the Adventist Health Study, those who ate nuts regularly experienced an extra 5.6 years of life expectancy free of heart disease compared to those who rarely ate nuts.

of the omega-3 fats in our diets (reviewed in chapter on fats). Eat nuts more often than seeds.

- Certain nuts are higher in certain nutrients. Almonds are particularly rich in vitamin E and magnesium. Peanuts are particularly rich in folate. Walnuts are rich in omega-3 fats (they're also rich in omega-6 fats). Hazelnuts are especially rich in vitamin E and copper. Cashews are rich in copper and magnesium. Brazil nuts are loaded with selenium. Pine nuts are higher in iron than other nuts. The least nutritious nut is the macadamia nut.

Moral of the story: eating a *variety* of nuts probably makes the most sense.

Sometimes I Feel Like a Nut

Six Easy Ways to Enjoy Nuts
(choose unsalted varieties more often)

1 Sprinkle on cereal.

2 Sprinkle on salads.

3 Enjoy with cooked veggies, rice or pasta.

4 Use in stir-fries.

5 Snack on them (portable and great for hectic days).

6 Eat a peanut butter sandwich (try with apple slices, lettuce, raisins, banana or even kiwi for something different).

THE ULTIMATE HEALTHY EATING PLAN

Enjoy 1/2 to 1 serving of nuts five times a week.

---

peanut butter

QUESTION OF THE DAY
"Should I buy natural peanut butter to avoid hydrogenated fats?" Contrary to popular belief, regular or homogenized peanut butters are very low in hydrogenated fats and therefore a healthy choice. Although they are slightly higher in sugar and sometimes salt, they have the advantage that they don't need to be stored in the fridge. The choice is yours. Most important, don't buy fat-reduced peanut butter. You get less of the healthy fats and save few, if any, calories.

FABULOUS FLAX

THE OBJECTIVES OF THE ULTIMATE HEALTHY EATING PLAN ARE TO REDUCE YOUR RISK OF DISEASE BY

optimizing

ground flaxseed

THE POWER OF FLAX

One of the greatest of all the medieval kings, King Charlemagne, considered the seeds of the flax plant so healthy he passed laws requiring their consumption. Today, Dr. Stephen Cunnane, a researcher at the University of Toronto, calls flax one of the most promising foods of the 21st century. These tasty, tiny, reddish-brown seeds contain a unique mix of fiber, beneficial plant compounds and heart-healthy fats, which appear to offer incredible protection against disease —especially heart disease and certain cancers.

Fabulous Fiber

Flaxseeds are an incredibly rich source of fiber. A mere 1/4 cup (50 mL) of ground flax contains 9 grams of fiber (wheat bran, often touted as the fiber all-star, contains about 6 grams of fiber per 1/4 cup (50 mL). Flax contains both soluble and insoluble fiber. While both types of fiber appear to play a role in protecting your heart, soluble fiber is especially important for lowering blood cholesterol levels. Several recent studies have reported lower levels of both total cholesterol and LDL cholesterol (the artery-clogging kind) in people who consume flax regularly. Soluble fiber also helps manage and prevent diabetes by keeping blood sugar levels in check. As for the health of your gastrointestinal tract, including regular bowel movements (yes, I do have to talk about the frequency of your bathroom visits!), it's the insoluble fiber in flax that's most helpful here.

QUESTION OF THE DAY
"Where do I buy flax?" As the awareness of the health benefits of flax increase, so does its availability. If you can't find it at your local supermarket (be sure to ask), it's widely available at health food stores and most bulk food stores.

Good-For-You Fats

Flaxseeds are by far the best food source of alpha-linolenic acid, the type of omega-3 fat found in plants that most of us need more of (this fat was also discussed in the Healthy-For-You-Fats chapter). Results from the Health Professionals Follow-Up Study, the Lyon Diet Health Study, the Multiple Risk Factor Intervention Trial and the Nurses' Health Study indicate that people who consume more alpha-linolenic acid are less likely to have a heart attack. If they do have a heart attack, they're also less likely to die from it. That's because alpha-linolenic acid helps your heart keep a strong and regular beat. Irregular heart beats (called arrhythmias) are a leading cause of heart attacks. Alpha-linolenic acid is also very important because your body converts some of it to EPA/DHA (the very beneficial fish form of omega-3 fats). This form of omega-3 fats has multiple health benefits including a reduction in risk of blood clots, some cancers, arthritis and more (all of this is discussed in detail in the Fantastic Fish chapter).

Cancer-Fighting Lignans

Flaxseeds are by far the best food source of beneficial plant compounds called lignans. Flaxseeds contain over 100 times more lignans than other lignan-containing foods such as vegetables, fruit and grains. Lignans are a type of plant compound with hormone-like activity (also referred to as phytoestrogens). They are especially important players in the fight against hormone-sensitive cancers like breast and prostate cancer. In preliminary research, animals fed flaxseed and injected with cancer cells did not form tumors. When tumors were already present, a diet rich in flaxseed caused the tumors to shrink. More recent human studies—particularly with breast cancer—have confirmed flax's cancer-protection potential. Lignans are thought to reduce cancer risk by influencing the production, availability and action of hormones. For example, by reducing the availability of estrogen, they block the development and spread of cancer cells (high blood levels of estrogen are thought to stimulate the growth of tumors).

Enjoying Flax

The Ultimate Healthy Eating Plan recommends consuming 1 to 2 servings of ground flaxseed most days of the week.

ONE SERVING	1 tablespoon (15 mL) of ground flaxseed

RESEARCH HIGHLIGHT
In a study from the University of Toronto, healthy women consuming flaxseed for four weeks significantly reduced total cholesterol and LDL or ("bad") cholesterol levels. They also experienced a significant increase in bowel movements (say farewell to constipation!).

RESEARCH HIGHLIGHT
In a study from Duke University Medical Center, eating flaxseed daily as part of a low-fat diet, significantly decreased the growth of cancer cells in men with prostate cancer.

Nine Important Flax Facts and Tips

1 Eat ground flax. Whole flaxseeds often pass through the gastrointestinal tract undigested.

2 Buy ground flax or grind it up yourself with a coffee grinder.

3 Whole flaxseed can be stored at room temperature for up to a year. Ground flaxseed can be stored in the fridge for about 4 months.

4 The easiest way to enjoy flax is to sprinkle it on your cereal each morning. You can also sprinkle it on yogurt, soups or salads. Mixing ground flax with a bit of honey or peanut butter and spreading it on whole-wheat toast is another tasty option.

5 There are four different recipes for muffins containing flax in this book. Each muffin contains 1 tablespoon (15 mL) of ground flax. Try them. They are outstanding!

6 Flax oil does not provide the same benefits as ground flax. It does not contain the health-protective plant lignans or fiber.

7 The flax content of store-bought flax breads or muffins varies widely. If you do buy them, choose products that contain ground flax combined with 100% whole grains such as whole-wheat flour (many products contain whole flax combined mostly with white flour).

8 Don't consume more than the recommended 1 to 2 servings of ground flaxseed daily. First, flax is a relatively concentrated source of calories. Each tablespoon (15 mL) of ground flaxseed contains 40 calories. Second, research on flax is still in the preliminary stages. Additional studies will further our understanding of the optimal amount of flax required for good health.

9 For more information on flax, including lots of recipes, visit www.flaxcouncil.ca.

THE ULTIMATE HEALTHY EATING PLAN

Enjoy 1 to 2 servings of ground flaxseed most days of the week.

RESEARCH HIGHLIGHT

In a study from the University of Toronto, a flaxseed muffin consumed daily by women diagnosed with breast cancer significantly slowed the growth of tumor cells. The results were similar (although not quite as strong) to taking the drug tamoxifen—a drug frequently prescribed for the prevention and treatment of breast cancer. Further research, including large-scale studies, will tell us more about the role of flax in the fight against breast cancer.

QUESTION OF THE DAY

"Which is better, brown flaxseed or golden flaxseed?" Some distributors of golden flaxseed claim it is nutritionally superior to brown flaxseed. Research from the Flax Council of Canada, however, indicates that both types are good choices and very similar in composition.

RESEARCH HIGHLIGHT

In a study from the University of Minnesota, premenopausal women fed flaxseed (about 1 rounded tablespoon) every day for two months showed a 31% improvement in the ratio of breast cancer-protective to breast cancer-promoting chemicals in their blood.

TIME FOR **TEA**

THE OBJECTIVES OF THE ULTIMATE HEALTHY EATING PLAN ARE TO REDUCE YOUR RISK OF DISEASE BY

optimizing

green tea | black tea
| fluids, including water

THE BEVERAGE QUESTION

What combination of beverages can best contribute to long-term health? This is a very interesting and important question. We know water is absolutely essential to good health. Name almost any major function of the human body and water plays a starring role. In fact, every living cell in our bodies depends on water to carry out its essential functions. We know that beverages like milk, vegetable juices and fruit juices also fit into a healthy diet. But what about coffee and tea? While drinking moderate amounts of coffee (about 2 to 3 cups daily) doesn't appear to be harmful to health, more and more research suggests that tea should be your beverage of choice.

Fabulous Flavonoids

A growing body of evidence suggests that moderate consumption of tea may protect against several forms of cancer and heart disease. Tea is a very rich source of plant compounds called flavonoids. Flavonoids appear to be important players in the disease-prevention game. They appear to help reduce the risk of disease by acting as potent antioxidants in the body. For example, by helping to put cell-damaging free radicals out of business, they help reduce the buildup of plaque on artery walls and stop the formation and spread of cancerous cells. The flavonoids in tea may also suppress the growth of harmful bacteria. In doing so, they help prevent the development of bacterial infections and even dental caries (cavities). Preliminary research also suggests a role for tea in the prevention of arthritis.

QUOTE OF THE DAY

"Tea cannot replace the nutritional value of fruits and vegetables, but it is a good complementary source of antioxidants."

Dr. John Weisburger, Chair of the 2nd International Symposium on Tea and Human Health

RESEARCH HIGHLIGHT

In animal studies, tea flavonoids inhibited the development of a variety of cancers including lung, esophageal, gastrointestinal and skin cancers. Very few other potential cancer-preventive agents have shown such strong activity in animal models in concentrations normally consumed by humans.

Tea appears to influence enzymes in the body that inhibit the growth and spread of abnormal cells. More studies are required in humans to better understand tea's role in the prevention of disease.

Green or Black?

Both green and black tea come from the same plant (the Camellia sinensis bush). The flavonoids they contain, however, are different due to the way they are processed (black tea is fermented, green is not). Green tea is especially rich in a flavonoid called epigallocatechin gallate (more frequently referred to as EGCG). Black tea is rich in flavonoids called thearubigens and theaflavins. The good news—all these flavonoids display antioxidant activity, and both green and black teas demonstrate the ability to fight disease. Is one better than the other? Overall, the research on tea is still in the preliminary stages. Research to date, however, suggests that green tea may offer greater disease protection—especially against cancer. Further research will tell us more.

Cup of Tea, Mate?

The Ultimate Healthy Eating Plan recommends drinking 3 to 6 cups of green or black tea each day. A typical cup of tea is 3/4 cup (175 mL). Based on the preliminary research to date, this amount is reasonable and may have a positive impact on health.

Things You Should Know About Tea

• Tea consumption can contribute significantly to the daily antioxidant requirements of humans. In a Tufts University study from Boston, the antioxidant capacity of tea leaves ranked number one in a list of 22 antioxidant-rich vegetables.

• A typical cup of tea contains about 40 mg of caffeine. That's roughly one-third to one-half of the amount found in a cup of brewed coffee. A moderate and safe amount of caffeine is considered to be about 300 mg per day. In other words, you could drink almost 8 cups of tea daily (if you didn't get caffeine from any other source) and still stay within the recommended limit. Choosing decaffeinated tea is always an option. However, most decaffeinated teas contain considerably less flavonoids—many about half as much as regular teas (some flavonoids are lost during processing).

• Herbal teas don't count towards your daily tea quota. They are primarily infusions of flowers, herbs or spices. While their compounds may have health-enhancing properties of their own, they do not provide the same disease-reducing benefits as green or black tea.

• If you like iced tea, make your own. When tea is processed into powdered or bottled liquid

RESEARCH HIGHLIGHT
In the Iowa Women's Study involving more than 35,000 women, those who drank 2 or more cups of black tea daily were 60% less likely to develop cancers of the urinary tract and 32% less likely to develop cancers of the digestive tract.

RESEARCH HIGHLIGHT
In the Rotterdam Study involving more than 3000 women, those who drank 1 to 2 cups of black tea daily had a 50% lower risk of severe atherosclerosis (buildup of plaque on artery walls). Women who drank more than 5 cups had the lowest risk.

RESEARCH HIGHLIGHT
In the Zutphen Elderly Study involving more than 500 men, those who drank 5 cups of tea or more daily had about a 70% lower risk of stroke.

form, the flavonoid content is often decreased.

- Tea decreases the absorption of iron from plant foods. Many women do not get enough iron in their diets. There are two solutions to this dilemma. First, enjoy tea between meals. Second, enjoy a fruit or vegetable rich in vitamin C at the same meal. Vitamin C enhances the absorption of iron. For example, enjoy a glass of orange juice with your morning cup of tea and bowl of cereal. Other vegetables and fruit rich in vitamin C include kiwi, red and green peppers, papaya, broccoli, strawberries and citrus fruits like grapefruit.

Water—The Forgotten Nutrient

The Ultimate Healthy Eating Plan recommends consuming 6 to 8 cups (1.5 to 2 L) of water or other fluids each day.

The importance of water is best illustrated by the fact that we can live for several weeks without food, but only a few days without water. Water makes up more than 70% of the body's tissues and plays a role in nearly every body function, from regulating temperature and cushioning joints to bringing oxygen and nutrients to the cells and removing waste from the body. Why 6 to 8 cups (1.5 to 2 L) a day? Replacement is the name of the game. All day long you lose water—as you breathe, when you perspire, each time you make a trip to the toilet. People who lead moderately active lifestyles lose about 6 to 8 cups (1.5 to 2 L) of water each day. For optimal health and well-being, that water must be replaced. Drinking lots of water or other fluids also helps prevent constipation and reduces the risk of kidney stones.

Meeting Your Six- to Eight-a-Day Quota

1 Make it a habit to carry water with you at all times.

2 Keep a bottle or pitcher of water with you at work to enjoy throughout the day. If it's there, you'll drink it! If it's not, you won't!

3 Every time you brush your teeth, drink a glass of water.

4 When dining out, always ask for water with your meal.

5 Fluids like juice, milk and soup all count towards your daily water quota. Most people easily consume at least half of their required fluid intake in this form.

6 Coffee and tea are mild diuretics, meaning they increase water loss. But they do still contribute to your water intake. Simply count each cup of tea or coffee as 1/2 cup of water.

drinking tea

GOOD ADVICE
Don't drink your tea scalding hot! While tea is generally linked to lower rates of disease, drinking your tea when it's very, very hot may increase your risk of cancer of the esophagus.

QUESTION OF THE DAY
"How long should I brew my tea to get the most antioxidants?" About 3 to 5 minutes—85% of the antioxidants are released within this time.

RESEARCH HIGHLIGHT
In a University of Toronto study involving over 1200 men, drinking more than 2 cups of tea per day was associated with a 30% decrease in the risk of prostate cancer.

7 For each alcoholic drink you consume, drink an extra glass of water. Alcohol is very dehydrating.

8 Drink extra water before, during and after physical activity.

9 Generally, both tap water and bottled water are safe choices. The downside of tap water is that it's chlorinated. Chlorine can react with organic material in fresh water and create a number of byproducts (called trihalomethanes) that have been linked to a small increased risk of some cancers. The downside of bottled water is the cost and the fact that most don't contain fluoride —an important nutrient for dental health. Some bottled mineral waters are also high in sodium.

THE ULTIMATE HEALTHY EATING PLAN

Enjoy 3 to 6 cups of green or black tea each day (a typical cup of tea is 3/4 cup/175mL). Enjoy 6 to 8 cups (1.5 to 2 L) of water or other fluids daily.

RESEARCH HIGHLIGHT
In a recent animal study, mice were injected with a substance that causes a condition similar to rheumatoid arthritis in people. They were then given either water or green tea (equivalent to a human drinking about 4 cups per day) as a regular part of their diet. In the green-tea group, less than half the mice developed arthritis, while in the water group, over 90% did. Further research will tell us more.

WHAT ABOUT **WINE**?

THE OBJECTIVES OF THE ULTIMATE HEALTHY EATING PLAN ARE TO REDUCE YOUR RISK OF DISEASE BY

moderating

alcohol | wine | beer | liquor

| if you choose to drink

OVERWHELMING EVIDENCE

The evidence is overwhelming! Based on over 40 studies from different populations around the world, people who consume alcohol in moderation significantly reduce their risk of heart disease. This is not a "maybe thing" or a "we need more research thing"—this is one of the most consistent findings of nutrition research to date. People who drink alcohol in moderation—no more than one drink a day for women and two drinks a day for men—reduce their risk of heart disease by 25% to 40% as compared to nondrinkers.

QUOTE OF THE DAY

"The evidence of a beneficial effect of alcohol is now massive."

Richard Doll, Professor of Medicine, Oxford

Heart-Healthy

How does alcohol help your heart? First, understand that all alcohol—wine, beer and liquor—is good for your heart, not just red wine, as commonly believed. It is the actual alcohol (also referred to as ethanol) in these beverages that is responsible for most of the heart-healthy benefits. Alcohol benefits the heart by increasing levels of HDL ("good") cholesterol in the blood. HDL helps carry cholesterol out of the bloodstream and back to the liver for disposal. The average HDL level of drinkers is 10% to 15% higher than that of nondrinkers (nothing else in your diet influences HDL in such a consistent manner). Alcohol also reduces the formation of potentially harmful blood clots. Many heart attacks and strokes are caused by blood clots forming in a partially blocked artery. Lastly, research also suggests that alcohol may help prevent inflammation of the artery wall and thereby help prevent the development of plaque or fatty deposits.

alcohol & heart disease

QUOTE OF THE DAY

"A large number of recent studies have consistently demonstrated a reduction in coronary heart disease with moderate consumption of alcohol. Any prohibition of alcohol would then deny such persons a potentially sizable health benefit."

Dr. Thomas Pearson, Nutrition Committee, American Heart Association

RESEARCH HIGHLIGHT

In a study by the American Cancer Society involving almost 500,000 men and women, the risk of heart disease was 30% to 40% lower in men and women who consumed one or more drinks daily. Overall, people who consumed one drink daily also lived the longest.

RESEARCH HIGHLIGHT

In the North Manhattan Stroke Study involving over 1800 men and women, those drinking up to 2 drinks per day had a significantly lower risk of stroke compared to nondrinkers. Heavy drinking (greater than 5 drinks per day) was associated with an increased risk of stroke.

The Red Wine Debate

In 1991, the television show *60 Minutes* aired a segment about the "French Paradox" and the possible benefits of drinking red wine. The following month, sales of red wine surged by 44% in the United States! If you choose to drink alcohol, should red wine be your beverage of choice? Red wine is as beneficial as other forms of alcohol and may provide some additional benefits. Red wine is particularly rich in a type of plant compound called flavonoids, which are also found in tea and various vegetables and fruit. Flavonoids also occur in other alcoholic beverages, such as dark beer. Some research suggests that these plant compounds, which appear to act as antioxidants in the body, provide additional benefits for heart health. For example, they may help prevent damage to the artery wall and help keep arteries relaxed or dilated. At this time, more research is required. Not all studies found that red wine offered an additional benefit when compared with other alcoholic beverages. Some researchers question whether the amount of flavonoids in red wine is enough to influence heart health significantly. Bottom line? If you currently drink red wine in moderation, enjoy it. We know the alcohol it contains is good for your heart, and maybe, just maybe, the plant compounds may provide additional benefits as well.

Your Daily Quota

If you choose to drink alcohol, the Ultimate Healthy Eating Plan recommends no more than one drink per day for women and no more than two drinks per day for men.

ONE DRINK	5 oz (145 mL) wine
	12 oz (350 mL) beer
	1.5 oz (45 mL) 80-proof spirits/liquor

QUOTE OF THE DAY
"There is no clear evidence that wine is more beneficial than other forms of alcohol, although further research is needed regarding the potential protective effects of substances unique to wine."

American Heart Association Science Advisory, January 2001

QUESTION OF THE DAY
"I don't usually drink alcohol during the week, but I tend to drink a lot on the weekends. Is this still beneficial for the heart?" For optimal heart health, drinking small amounts of alcohol regularly and with meals appears to offer the best protection—especially for reducing the risk of blood clots. Consuming 4 or 5 drinks within 4 hours (common weekend social drinking for many people) is associated with an increased risk of stroke—especially for people who are already at high risk for stroke.

An Important Note of Caution

Before you rush out to your local liquor or beer store, please be aware of the following:

1 You don't need alcohol to be healthy. A diet rich in foods like whole grains, beans, nuts, fish, vegetables and fruit provides excellent protection against disease (without any risks!).

2 The benefits of consuming alcohol apply only when it is consumed in moderation. Beyond that, excess consumption is a major contributor to death and disability. People who regularly drink in excess cause significant damage to their heart and liver and are at increased risk for various cancers. They are also at much greater risk for accidents and injuries.

3 For women, alcohol consumed even in moderation (one drink per day) is associated with significantly higher rates of breast cancer. If you have a family history of breast cancer, research suggests you abstain from alcohol or limit your consumption to no more than one to two drinks per week. A diet rich in folate (folic acid) also appears to reduce the risk of breast cancer in women who consume alcohol. Folate-rich foods include asparagus, spinach, broccoli, orange juice, beans, fortified cereals and peanuts.

4 Alcohol is an addictive substance. No one can predict who will suffer from alcoholism or when someone will cross the line.

5 You don't have to drink alcohol every day to experience the health benefits. Even just 1 to 2 drinks per week are associated with lower rates of heart disease and stroke.

6 Alcohol provides the greatest benefit to people who are middle-aged and older—the time when the risk of heart disease is greatest. For most young adults, the risks of consuming alcohol outweigh the benefits.

7 If you want to manage your waistline, watch your alcohol intake. Drink alcohol only in moderate amounts and be careful of alcohol's ability to rev up your appetite. One study found that having 1 alcoholic drink before a meal caused people to eat on average an extra 200 calories from food—this on top of the added calories that come from the drink itself.

THE ULTIMATE HEALTHY EATING PLAN

If you choose to drink alcohol (wine, beer, liquor), women should consume no more than 1 drink and men no more than 2 drinks each day.

RESEARCH HIGHLIGHT
In addition to alcohol providing benefits for your heart, preliminary research suggests that the moderate consumption of alcohol may also reduce your risk of osteoporosis, macular degeneration (the leading cause of blindness in older age), diabetes and possibly dementia (mental decline).

RESEARCH HIGHLIGHT
A study of more than 3500 Japanese-American men aged 71 to 93 showed that those who drank moderately throughout middle age performed better on tests of mental ability. The heaviest drinkers in the study had the poorest test performances.

QUOTE OF THE DAY
"An individual's risk for developing alcoholism is difficult, if not impossible, to determine."
American Heart Association Science Advisory, January 2001

LEAVING ROOM
FOR **CHOCOLATE**

THE OBJECTIVES OF THE ULTIMATE HEALTHY EATING PLAN ARE TO ENCOURAGE CHOCOLATE-LOVERS TO

enjoy

chocolate in small quantities to make
healthy foods taste better

choose

certain types of chocolate containing
higher amounts of beneficial plant
compounds more often

CHOCOHOLICS UNITE!

There's food—and then there's chocolate. Based on a North American study, chocolate is craved by more people (especially women) than any other food. Seventy-five percent of chocolate-cravers also claim that when they have a yearning for chocolate, no other food will do. The sensory reward of chocolate is exceptional—the sweet aroma, the melt-in-your-mouth texture and the wonderful, rich flavor. But could this food, which is also very high in fat and calories, possibly have a place in a healthy diet?

Further Research Will Tell Us More

The research on chocolate is still in the preliminary stages. Here's what we do know. The cocoa bean (from which chocolate and cocoa are made) is extremely rich in plant compounds called flavonoids. Flavonoids are also found in tea, red wine and certain vegetables and fruit. They appear to protect health in part by acting as antioxidants and preventing damage to body cells that leads to disease. The cocoa bean is unique in that it contains very high quantities of flavonoids called procyanidins (apples are also rich in procyanidins—most of which are in the skin). Procyanidins are made up of several flavonoid units joined together. In preliminary research, it is the larger flavonoids that appear to demonstrate greater antioxidant potential.

QUOTE OF THE DAY
"If you are not feeling well, if you have not slept, chocolate will revive you. But you have no chocolate pot! I think of that again and again. How will you manage?"

Marquise de Sevigne (letter written by a mother to her daughter in 1671, a time when chocolate was already adored by many)

QUOTE OF THE DAY
"Chocolate cravings are real."

Journal of the American Dietetic Association, October 1999

Heart Healthy?

In preliminary research, chocolate flavonoids may help protect the heart by

- preventing damage to LDL ("bad") cholesterol (when LDL becomes damaged or oxidized it is more likely to result in the formation of plaque on the artery wall)

- reducing platelet aggregation and adhesion (reducing the risk of plaque buildup on artery walls and the risk of blood clots)

- relaxing the inner surface of blood vessel walls

Not All Chocolate Is Created Equal

The Ultimate Healthy Eating Plan recommends choosing chocolate that contains higher amounts of flavonoids more often (if you like chocolate, that is!).

Dark chocolate generally contains about three times the amount of flavonoids as milk chocolate. White chocolate does not contain any. The way in which chocolate or cocoa is processed, however, is what's really critical. Manufacturing processes, such as fermentation and roasting of the cocoa bean, often destroy many of the flavonoids present. Mars Incorporated, the makers of products such as M&M's, is currently the only large, North American company to communicate to the consumer that they process their chocolate so as to maximize the retention of naturally occurring cocoa flavonoids. Many of their products now carry the Cocoapro logo to help communicate this message. Much of the chocolate research to date has been done using either the Mars Dove Dark Chocolate Bar or M&M's Semi-Sweet Baking Bits. Therefore, at this time, I recommend choosing products such as the Dove Dark Bar (only available in the United States) or M&M's Chocolate Candies, and using M&M's Semi-Sweet Baking Bits in your recipes (including the recipes in this book that call for chocolate chips) more often. As more research unfolds, we may ultimately see a day when all companies list the flavonoid content of their chocolate on the label.

RESEARCH HIGHLIGHT
In the ORAC test—considered the gold standard for measuring the antioxidant power of foods—a dark chocolate bar and a milk chocolate bar scored much higher than black tea, green tea or 1/2 cup (125 mL) of blueberries.

RESEARCH HIGHLIGHT
In a recent study from the University of California, the consumption of flavonoid-rich chocolate (slightly less than 1 ounce or 25 grams of M&M's semi-sweet baking pieces) was associated with a marked decrease in platelet aggregation and activation (stickiness of the blood). Both platelet aggregation and adhesion are associated with a higher risk of plaque formation on the artery wall and an increased potential of the blood to clot.

Fat and Calorie Overload!

Please don't misinterpret my message. This chapter is not a permission slip to load up on chocolate. Don't believe (not even for a minute!) that chocolate will ever take the place of healthy, disease-fighting foods like vegetables and fruit—not even close. Chocolate is a food with potential health benefits (the research is still in the early stages) and should be enjoyed primarily because you love it. It's also a food that comes with a heavy price tag—lots of calories and fat in a small package. Much of the fat is also the saturated kind, the type we need to eat less of, not more.

Satisfying Your Craving Without Sacrificing Your Waistline

The Ultimate Healthy Eating Plan recommends enjoying chocolate in small quantities to make healthy foods taste better.

Here Are Some Chocolatey Examples

- Low-fat chocolate milk is a favorite with adults and kids alike. Save calories by making your own (use about 1 tsp/5 mL chocolate syrup or powder per serving). Ready-made, store-bought chocolate milk often contains double the calories.

- Enjoy chocolate-flavored soy milk. Better yet, try our Super Chocolate Banana Soy Shake (page 245).

- Low-fat chocolate pudding makes a great snack. It's also a fun dip. Serve it to kids with fresh fruit.

- Add a few chocolate chips (or M&M's) to trail mix, whole-grain pancakes or whole-grain muffins.

- Dip strawberries or other fresh fruit into a bit of melted dark chocolate as a special treat at the end of a meal.

- Drizzle a teaspoon or two of chocolate syrup over a scoop of low-fat frozen yogurt.

- Enjoy a small serving of chocolate-covered nuts. Limit serving size to 1/2 ounce (14 g)—for example, 16 chocolate-covered peanuts or 12 chocolate-covered almonds.

- Enjoy chocolate-covered raisins. Limit serving to about 16.

If you do eat chocolate on its own or in less healthy foods like cookies, limit your serving to no more than about 75 calories and less than 5 grams fat each day.

chocolate & caffeine

QUESTION OF THE DAY

"Isn't chocolate high in caffeine?" A milk chocolate bar (1.8-oz / 50-g bar) contains anywhere from 2 to 30 mg of caffeine. A dark chocolate bar (1.8-oz / 50-g bar) contains anywhere from 10 to 60 mg of caffeine. A glass of chocolate milk generally contains less than 5 mg of caffeine—about the same as a cup of decaffeinated coffee. Current research supports limiting caffeine to about 300 mg daily. Bottom line: the caffeine content of chocolate should not be of concern when it's consumed in small amounts as part of a healthy diet.

GOOD ADVICE

If you find it difficult to consume chocolate without overindulging, consider avoiding chocolate altogether or limiting yourself to a once-a-week chocolate treat.

ONE SERVING OF CHOCOLATE	50 mini M&M's Chocolate Candies (1/2 of 1-oz/30-g tube)
	20 regular size M&M's Chocolate Candies
	2 to 3 squares (1/2 oz/14 g) of a typical chocolate bar
	1 Two-Bite Brownie (small brownie available in many supermarkets)
	6 Snackwell's Bite Size Chocolate Overload Cookies
	1 Snackwell Chocolatey Sandwich Cookie
	12 Chocolate Teddy Grahams

Remember that for most people just a taste or two of chocolate is often just as satisfying (and certainly better for the waistline) than a full-fledged chocolate binge.

THE ULTIMATE HEALTHY EATING PLAN

If you love chocolate, enjoy it primarily in small quantities to make healthy foods taste better. Choose mostly chocolate that contains higher amounts of flavonoids, such as M&M's Chocolate Candies.

THE **NUTRITIONAL**
SUPPLEMENT DEBATE

THE OBJECTIVES OF THE ULTIMATE HEALTHY EATING PLAN ARE TO REDUCE YOUR RISK OF DISEASE BY

ensuring

that your needs for all vitamins
and minerals are met

optimizing

vitamins and minerals linked to
a lower risk of disease

LET FOOD BE THY MEDICINE

If you'd like to roll out of bed each morning and pop a magic pill—a pill that promises optimal health, eternal youth and protection from disease—you're not alone. I have good news and bad. First, the good. You can dramatically influence your health, your risk of disease, your longevity and the overall quality of your life. The bad news: You're not going to do it with a pill. For ultimate health, you need food, glorious food (and an active lifestyle). The complex, disease-protective power of nutrient-rich, fiber-rich, omega-3-rich, antioxidant-rich and plant-compound-rich foods like vegetables, fruit, beans, fish, flax, nuts and whole grains just can't be beat.

The question is, can a pill or supplement assist you, along with your healthy diet, in your quest for a healthy life?

Make It a Multi

The Ultimate Healthy Eating Plan recommends taking a multivitamin and mineral supplement each day—especially if you are female or over the age of 50.

Best Eight Reasons to Pop a Multi

1 Inexpensive Insurance

Although the Ultimate Healthy Eating Plan was developed to optimize your intake of all essential nutrients, taking a multivitamin pill is a low-cost and easy way to help make sure this goal is met—especially on the days when you don't quite manage to follow the plan.

2 Do No Harm

Taking a multivitamin, rather than high doses of individual vitamins, is definitely your safest option when it comes to supplements. Vitamins and minerals interact with one another in a very delicate balance. Too much of one nutrient can interfere with the absorption and use of another nutrient.

QUOTE OF THE DAY
"Whole natural foods harbor a whole ratatouille of compounds that have never seen the inside of a vitamin bottle for the simple reason that scientists have not until very recently even known they existed, let alone brewed them into pills."

Newsweek

For example, too much zinc interferes with the absorption of both copper and iron. And too much beta-carotene can affect blood levels of lycopene. Many nutrients are also toxic when taken in high doses—especially vitamin A, vitamin B6, vitamin D, iron, zinc and selenium. Lastly, many nutrients work synergistically in the body (they work best together). For example, the B vitamins work as a team, as do many of the antioxidant vitamins such as vitamin E and selenium.

3 Women Need It

Iron deficiency is the most common nutrient deficiency among women of childbearing age. Even mild iron deficiency is linked to impaired learning ability, reduced work performance and a lower resistance to infections. Prior to menopause, women have higher requirements for iron because they lose significant amounts of iron each month during their period. Getting enough iron from food can be a challenge, especially if red meat is not a major part of your diet (as is the case with the Ultimate Healthy Eating Plan). That's why a multi makes sense.

4 Over Fifty

Research shows that your ability to absorb or utilize certain nutrients decreases as you get older. For example, due to decreases in gastric acid secretion,

as many as 30% of older adults are unable to absorb vitamin B12 in the form that it's naturally found in food (bound to protein). That's why the most recent nutrient recommendations from the National Academy of Sciences now state that adults age 51 years of age and older should obtain the majority of their vitamin B12 from a supplement or from a food (such as soy milk) to which vitamin B12 has been added. As we get older, many of us (depending on our activity level) also eat less food in order to manage our waistlines. Less food means less nutrition and a greater chance that nutrient needs will not be met.

5 Disease-Fighting Folic Acid

Folic acid (referred to as folate when it occurs naturally in food) is definitely considered a super hero in the disease prevention world. When consumed by women just before and during pregnancy, it can prevent devastating birth defects involving brain and nerve disorders. It appears to reduce the risk of heart disease by decreasing levels of a compound in the blood called homocysteine. Homocysteine appears to increase the risk of heart disease by damaging artery walls and increasing the risk of blood clots (vitamin B6 and B12 are also important for healthy homocysteine levels). Folic acid is linked to significantly lower rates of cancer, including cancer of the colon. It's critical

women

RESEARCH HIGHLIGHT
In the Nurses' Health Study involving about 80,000 women, those with the highest intakes of folic acid and vitamin B6 were 45% less likely to suffer from heart disease. For many of these women, a multivitamin supplement was a key contributor to their higher intakes of these nutrients.

RESEARCH HIGHLIGHT
In the Nurses' Health Study involving about 80,000 women, those who had been taking a multivitamin for 15 years were 75% less likely to develop cancer of the colon. Folic acid was identified as the key nutrient in multivitamins responsible for this major reduction in risk.

for the healthy development of DNA—the blueprint your cells use to reproduce.

While the Ultimate Healthy Eating Plan optimizes your folate intake through foods like dark green and orange veggies and fruit, beans and whole grains, a multivitamin containing this nutrient is recommended for three reasons. First, getting enough folic acid is a challenge even when consuming a healthy diet. Second, folic acid in a supplement (the synthetic form) is much better absorbed by your body (about 30% to 50% better) than the form found in food. Third, some researchers suggest that for optimal disease prevention, especially for heart-disease prevention, you may be wise to consume higher amounts of this nutrient. The current recommendation is 400 mcg per day. Some researchers suggest closer to 600 mcg may be ideal. Bottom line: this is a very important nutrient and taking a multi ensures you're getting enough.

6 Hard-to-Get Vitamin D

Getting enough vitamin D is essential for the optimal absorption of calcium in your diet. Vitamin D may also help reduce the risk of some cancers, including breast, prostate and colon cancer. If, however, you don't drink two glasses of milk each day (or soy milk fortified with vitamin D) as recommended in the Plan, it's unlikely you'll meet your needs for this important nutrient. This is especially true if you live in a northern location such as Canada (vitamin D is made by your body when sunlight strikes your skin). Beyond the age of 50, your need for vitamin D increases significantly.

7 Other Hard-to-Get-Nutrients

In addition to providing iron, folic acid and vitamin D, a multivitamin helps boost your intake of other nutrients that are also often challenging to get and yet are very important to good health. These include zinc, copper, magnesium and vitamin E.

8 Protection from Disease

Preliminary research suggests that people who regularly take a multivitamin may reduce their risk of heart disease, cancer (especially colon cancer) and cataracts. A multi may also help keep your immune system healthy—especially as you get older.

Three Top Tips for Choosing a Multi

1 Cover all the bases. Choose a multi that contains a complete mix of vitamins and minerals. Some of the specialty formulas for women, for example, are higher in calcium, but contain only a handful of other minerals. The most complete formulas contain 29 essential vitamins and minerals.

women & men

RESEARCH HIGHLIGHT

In a study from the University of Wisconsin-Madison Medical School involving more than 3000 people aged 43 to 86, those who took a multivitamin for more than 10 years had a 60% lower risk of developing cataracts.

QUESTION OF THE DAY

"I've heard that men and older women should not take supplements containing iron. Is this true?" While women of childbearing age often don't get enough iron due to losses from menstruation, post-menopausal women and men may want to consider a formula that is lower in iron, such as Centrum Select or similar brands. These groups generally do not need extra iron and there is some evidence that excess iron may increase the risk of heart disease by causing damage to artery walls.

2 Save your money. It's okay to buy store-brand and generic products. They still do the job.

3 Use the chart on the next page to choose a multi that best suits your nutrient needs. Keep in mind that certain minerals such as calcium and magnesium are too bulky for a single multivitamin to contain 100% of your daily requirement. Be especially sure to choose a multi that best meets your needs for folic acid, iron and vitamin D, as well as the antioxidant vitamins—vitamin E, vitamin C and selenium.

Antioxidant All-Stars?

The Ultimate Healthy Eating Plan does not recommend taking high doses of antioxidant vitamins, with the possible exception of vitamin E. If you choose to take vitamin E, take no more than 100 to 400 IU per day.

Certain nutrients, including vitamin C, vitamin E, beta-carotene and selenium are believed to act as antioxidants within the body. Antioxidants' "claim to fame" is their ability to significantly reduce the risk of disease and even slow down the aging process by stopping nasty free radicals from damaging body cells. While it's clear that eating foods rich in antioxidants—like vegetables and fruit—helps prevent diseases like heart disease,

cancer and cataracts, the link between high doses of antioxidant supplements and disease has not been conclusively shown. My recommendations are as follows:

Vitamin C

The recommended intake for vitamin C is 75 mg/day for women and 90 mg/day for men. Some researchers suggest 200 mg/day is optimal to saturate body tissues. The most promising research links vitamin C supplements to the prevention of cataracts. Bottom line: as long as your diet is rich in vegetables and fruit (at least 5 servings a day), it's easy to meet your needs for this nutrient through food.

Vitamin E

The recommended intake for vitamin E is 22 IU of natural source vitamin E (or 33 IU of the synthetic form). Of all the antioxidants, vitamin E supplements have demonstrated the most promise in terms of disease prevention. Vitamin E supplements have been linked to lower rates of heart disease, prostate and colon cancer, arthritis, Parkinson's disease, diabetes and Alzheimer's disease. Having said that, much of the research has been either inconclusive or preliminary. It's also important to note that the largest study involving over 9000 people at high risk for heart

build immunity

RESEARCH HIGHLIGHT

A number of studies have reported a positive link between multivitamin use and immune function. In a 12-month study, the average number of days of illness due to infection was 23 for those who received supplements versus 48 for those who did not.

QUESTION OF THE DAY

"When is the best time to take a multivitamin?" To get the most out of your multi, take it with meals and drink some fluids to help it dissolve.

NUTRIENT	RECOMMENDED DAILY INTAKE	UPPER SAFE LIMIT
Vitamin A	Women **700 mcg** / Men **900 mcg** (Women **2300 IU** / Men **3000 IU**)	3000 mcg (10,000 IU)
Beta-carotene	none determined (research suggests that the upper safe limit is about 9 mg/15,000 IU)	none determined
Vitamin E	15 mg (22 IU)	1000 mg (1500 IU)
Vitamin C	Women **75 mg** / Men **90 mg**	2000 mg
Folic Acid (folate)	400 mcg	1000 mcg
Thiamin (vitamin B1)	Women **1.1 mg** / Men **1.2 mg**	none determined
Riboflavin (vitamin B2)	Women **1.1 mg** / Men **1.3 mg**	none determined
Niacin	Women **14 mg** / Men **16 mg**	35 mg
Pyridoxine (vitamin B6) over age 50	1.3 mg Women **1.5 mg** / Men **1.7 mg**	100 mg
Vitamin B12	2.4 mcg (over age 50, take in the form of a supplement)	none determined
Vitamin D over age 50 over age 70	5 mcg (200 IU) 10 mcg (400 IU) 15 mcg (600 IU)	50 mcg (2000 IU)
Biotin	30 mcg	none determined
Pantothenic Acid	5 mg	none determined
Calcium over age 50	1000 mg 1200 mg	2500 mg
Phosphorus	700 mg	4000 mg
Iodine	150 mcg	1100 mg
Iron over age 50	Women **18 mg** / Men **8 mg** 8 mg	45 mg
Magnesium age 19 to 30 over age 31	Women **310 mg** / Men **400 mg** Women **320 mg** / Men **420 mg**	350 mg (the upper safe limit for magnesium only applies to intake from a supplement and does not include intake from food and water)

chart continued on next page

NUTRIENT	RECOMMENDED DAILY INTAKE	UPPER SAFE LIMIT
Copper	900 mcg	10,000 mcg
Manganese	Women 1.8 mg / Men 2.3 mg	11 mg
Chromium	Women 25 mcg / Men 35 mcg	none determined
Molybdenum	45 mcg	2000 mcg
Selenium	55 mcg	400 mcg
Zinc	Women 8 mg / Men 11 mg	40 mg
Choline	Women 425 mg / Men 550 mg	3500 mg

Source: National Academy of Sciences, Dietary Reference Intakes

Please note
The nutrient recommendations listed in this chart are for adults over 18 years old. Researchers feel there is currently not enough data to give recommended intakes for vitamin K, chromium, manganese, biotin, pantothenic acid and choline. Therefore, the numbers provided in this chart for these nutrients are based on average intakes for most healthy adults.

disease—the HOPE study (Heart Outcomes Prevention Evaluation Study)—reported no benefit from taking vitamin E supplements. Bottom line: it's challenging to meet current recommended intakes for vitamin E intake through food since you have to consume lots of nuts, seeds, vegetable oils and margarine. In addition, much of the research suggests that for optimal protection from disease higher amounts of vitamin E are required. You have two options. Option #1: Take a vitamin E supplement containing 100 to 400 IU of vitamin E. Option #2: Wait for more research, follow the Plan and take your daily multivitamin to ensure current recommendations for this nutrient are met.

RESEARCH HIGHLIGHT
A report prepared by the National Academy of Sciences involving more than 40 leading researchers concluded that there is insufficient evidence to support claims that taking megadoses of dietary antioxidants, such as selenium and vitamins C and E or carotenoids, including beta-carotene, can prevent chronic diseases. Furthermore, extremely large doses may actually lead to health problems.

Beta-carotene

Get your beta-carotene by eating lots of dark green and orange vegetables and fruit—not by taking a high-dose supplement. In a large Finnish study involving 29,000 male smokers, the risk of lung cancer was increased 18% in those taking high-dose supplements of beta-carotene. Subsequent studies showed similar results.

Selenium

The recommended intake for this nutrient is 55 mcg daily. Preliminary research suggests that taking 200 mcg in a supplement may significantly decrease the risk of some cancers, including cancer of the prostate, lung and colon. Never take more than 400 mcg; selenium is very toxic at high doses. Bottom line: the research on selenium is in the early stages. Large-scale studies are now underway that will help us understand its potential benefits. In the meantime, follow the Plan and take your multi. Selenium is found in whole grains, nuts, seafood, beans and poultry (all foods that are part of the Plan).

What About Calcium?

If you are following the Plan and consuming at least 3 to 4 servings of milk products or products fortified with calcium (such as soy milk) each day, a calcium supplement is not required. If you're unable to meet this requirement, consider a supplement. Calcium carbonate (such as is found in Tums) is the least expensive form of supplemental calcium. Take it with meals and take no more than 500 mg at a time for maximum absorption. Be sure to take your multivitamin for vitamin D.

THE ULTIMATE HEALTHY EATING PLAN

Take a multivitamin each day. Do not take high doses of antioxidant vitamins with the possible exception of vitamin E. If you choose to take vitamin E, take 100 to 400 IU daily.

ACTIVE LIVING
FOR A LIFETIME

THE OBJECTIVES OF THE ULTIMATE HEALTHY EATING PLAN ARE TO

make

physical activity, including both lifestyle
activities and regular planned exercise, a
regular part of your daily life

optimize

the amount and type of exercise you do
in order to reduce your risk of disease
and help you achieve and maintain a
healthy body weight

PARTICIPATION—NOT OPTIONAL!

Do you remember the vegetable and fruit chapter—the part where I wanted to jump, yell and do triple back-flips just to be sure you were paying attention? Guess what? I'm back! Ready to scream, sing, dance from the rooftops and generally do whatever it takes to communicate a message I know you've heard a million times (maybe a trillion zillion times!). Regular physical activity is essential (I'm talking critical, fundamental and so very, very important!) to good health.

Made to Move

Our bodies were built to move. When you're physically active, you live longer. You will also have a less bumpy, more enjoyable ride along the way. You significantly reduce your risk of heart disease, Type II diabetes, high blood pressure, osteoporosis and cancers of the colon and breast. You help keep your brain healthy and reduce your risk of diseases like Alzheimer's. You fall asleep faster and sleep more soundly. You smile more. You're much more likely to maintain a healthy weight. And if you lose weight, regular activity gets the highest score for helping to keep the weight off. Bottom line: an active and fit lifestyle (along with a healthy diet) is the greatest gift you can give yourself.

Take the Stairs

The Ultimate Healthy Eating Plan recommends increasing the amount of time and energy spent in activities of daily living.

QUOTE OF THE DAY
"If exercise were a drug, it would be the most prescribed medicine in the world."

National Institute of Aging

It's almost unavoidable to be lazy. We live in an environment in which it's much easier to sit than to move. We drive, we don't walk. We take elevators, not stairs. Many of us spend endless hours at jobs that require moving little more than the computer mouse. We have remotes or timers for everything from garage doors to TVs to coffee machines. Why, it even takes less energy to fluff a duvet than to make a bed. We live in an environment that's completely opposite of the one that shaped human evolution and optimizes good health. The solution? We have to build activity back into our lives.

Top Twelve Easy Ways to Build Activity Into Everyday Life

1 If you see stairs, take them. Pretend you have a serious allergy to elevators and escalators. If you live or work on the twenty-third floor, consider taking the stairs for three flights each day and an elevator for the rest of the ride.

2 Don't spend 15 minutes circling the parking lot looking for the spot closest to the door of the mall or supermarket. Park farther away and walk.

3 Put on loud music in your house and dance, dance, dance. (Singing loudly is also an option.) Dance with your family. Dance by yourself. Dancing is incredibly fun and good for the soul.

4 Keep the car in the driveway and walk. Walk to the corner store. Walk to the mailbox. Walk to the restaurant. Get off your bus one stop early and walk home.

5 Smile and say to yourself with enthusiasm, "I just love cleaning my house." Then vacuum that rug. Dust those shelves. Clean those toilet bowls. (Okay, forget the smile for the toilet bowls.)

6 Have a great garden. Spend time in your garden —planting, weeding, watering and pruning.

7 Cut your grass (but not by riding on top of a giant lawnmower!).

8 Shovel your driveway.

9 When you go grocery shopping, walk up and down every single aisle.

10 When watching your kid's soccer or hockey game, walk around the field or the arena at least two to three times.

11 Wear or take walking shoes with you to work. Have walking meetings. Take "three-minute mini walking breaks" around the office each hour. Go for a walk at lunch—even if it's only for five or ten minutes.

activity and health

QUOTE OF THE DAY
"Inactivity is about the same risk factor as smoking in terms of health."

Allan Rock,
Minister of Health, Canada

RESEARCH HIGHLIGHT
In a Swedish study involving 7000 men either diagnosed with Type II diabetes or considered at high risk for developing the disease, more than half of those who lost weight and became more physically active were able to reverse their resistance to insulin.

QUOTE OF THE DAY
"The only long-term way to control weight is to have a long-term regular physical activity program."

Dr. Gerald Fletcher,
Mayo Clinic

12 Don't get too comfortable on that couch! Cut back on sitting-down time and TV time. Clean out a closet. Call a friend with your portable telephone and walk while you talk. Play a game like Twister. If you must watch TV, use commercial time to do a few sit-ups, push-ups or simply to stretch that body of yours.

Each and every time you do one of these activities, give yourself a huge, big pat on the back. It all adds up and it really makes a difference!

Put It in Your Calendar (Then Do It!)

For optimal health, including disease-risk reduction, weight loss and weight maintenance, the Ultimate Healthy Eating Plan recommends a minimum of 30 minutes, and, ideally, 45 minutes to 1 hour, of planned, moderate-intensity physical activity on most and preferably all days of the week.

Top Eight Tips for "Planned" Activity

1 If you lack motivation, start by making a list (the longer the better!) of all the reasons that moving your body is well worth the effort. Focus on that list—especially on the days when your willpower is severely lacking. One woman found it motivating to hang a little black dress in front of her treadmill. Another man committed to being able to run a marathon by the end of the year. Figure out what motivates you.

2 Commit to working out regularly for at least a 3- to 6-month stretch. Many people find that after six months they're hooked for life. It becomes a habit that feels too good to give up.

3 Determine what activities you enjoy most and which ones fit most easily into your lifestyle. Men tend to like organized sports like hockey. Women, especially women with children, tend to prefer activities such as walking that are convenient and close to home.

4 Take 5 to 10 minutes at the beginning of each week to plan (even if it's just a rough plan) which activities you'll do each day. For example, Monday you'll go for a 45-minute walk after dinner and Tuesday you'll take a step class at the gym. By putting the activity into your calendar the chance of it actually happening is significantly increased! Plan longer workouts for the weekends when you usually have more time. If you find it difficult to plan a week's worth of activities, at least take a moment at the end of each day to decide what you are going to do the following day.

RESEARCH HIGHLIGHT

What do 3000 people who have lost an average of 60 pounds (27 kg) and kept if off for an average of five years have in common? Based on data from the National Weight Control Registry in the United States, they follow a high-carbohydrate, low-fat diet. They weigh themselves frequently and record what they eat on a regular basis in order to catch weight fluctuations early and act to correct them. Most important, they burn about 2700 calories a week in physical activity—the equivalent of about one hour of moderately intense activity every day. Moral of the story: you've got to move it to lose it!

RESEARCH HIGHLIGHT

Get fit! Researchers from the Cooper Institute in Dallas looked at the fitness habits of over 21,000 men. They found that men who were fit but overweight had a lower death rate than men who were lean but unfit. Men who were fit and lean had the lowest risk of death of all.

5 You don't have to do all of your planned exercise at the same time. For example, you could walk for half an hour in the morning before work and then go for another 15 to 30 minute walk after dinner.

6 Make working out fun. Listen to great music. Listen to motivational tapes or books on tape. Exercise with friends. Get a dog and walk it!

7 If you're going to join a health club, pick a good one. The extra money is usually well worth it. If you're new to the health club scene, take the beginner and orientation classes. (Taking an advanced step class on your first day is not a good idea!) Booking a few sessions with a personal trainer is also a super way to get started.

8 If you're going to purchase exercise equipment for your home, consider a good-quality treadmill (it's most likely to be used for the long term) plus some weights. Exercise videos are also very convenient and highly recommended. To order a great catalogue of exercise videos phone Collage Video at 1-800-433-6769. Some of my favorite instructors are Gin Miller, Kathy Smith and Kari Anderson.

Recommended Activities

The Ultimate Healthy Eating Plan recommends brisk walking and resistance exercises (lifting weights).

1 Walk This Way

Brisk walking is so easy. It's extremely convenient. And most people really enjoy it. It also offers tremendous health benefits. Research shows walking can reduce the risk of heart attack as much as vigorous exercises such as jogging, biking and swimming. In the Nurses' Health Study, women who walked briskly for 3 hours each week reduced their risk of a heart attack by 30% to 40%. Those who walked briskly for 5 hours or more each week cut their heart attack risk by about half. Just remember, I did say brisk walking, not leisurely stroll.

2 Lift It

You have more than 600 muscles throughout your body. Every move you make involves muscles. Resistance exercise (working out with weights) builds muscular strength and endurance. It's good for your heart; it helps keep your bones healthy and your mood lifted. Pound for pound, muscle also burns three times more calories than does just fat to sustain itself. This means the more muscle mass you have, the more efficiently and quickly you burn calories, even at rest. As you get older, you can lose up to half a pound (0.25 kg) of muscle

RESEARCH HIGHLIGHT
In a recent study from Duke University Medical Center, people suffering from depression were put either on a regular exercise program or treated with the antidepressant Zoloft. Not only did exercise work just as well at reducing or eliminating symptoms of depression, it did a better job than medication of preventing the depression from returning.

GOOD ADVICE
Setting fitness goals and monitoring your progress is a great way to fuel your motivation to stay active. Buy a pedometer from your local sporting goods store (ask the staff which model they recommend). It's a wonderful little gadget that clips on the waist of your pants and calculates how many steps you take each day. Aim for a minimum of 7000 steps each day and ideally 10,000 steps or more.

RESEARCH HIGHLIGHT
A study from the San Francisco Veterans Administration Medical Center involving about 6000 women reported that exercise keeps your mind sharp as you age. The decline in cognitive skills (thinking skills) was about 40% less in the women who were most active.

mass a year if you don't keep your muscles challenged. The result is middle-age waistline expansion (also referred to as middle-age spread). Aim for at least one and ideally two to three sessions per week. Get a demonstration video or work with a personal trainer to make sure you're using proper technique.

We Owe It To Our Children

We owe it to our children to keep them active. At a recent International Obesity Conference, researcher Professor Seideel said, "How we deal with childhood obesity is the biggest single public health challenge of this century." The waistlines of children around the world are expanding at an alarming rate. For the first time in history, record numbers of overweight children are being diagnosed with Type II diabetes as early as age 10 (this is a disease that typically hits closer to age 45 or 50). Sedentary lifestyles and poor diets are to blame. As a parent, I believe you not only can make a difference, you also have a responsibility to do so.

Keep Kids Moving Tips

1 Limit total computer time and TV time to about 1 hour and no more than 2 hours daily.

2 Make family time active time. Go to the playground, go biking, go skiing, go hiking.

3 Encourage your children to learn a variety of different sports such as swimming, soccer, baseball and skating. They'll be much more likely to carry these skills with them into adulthood and stay active.

4 Monkey see, monkey do. Children of active parents are much more likely to be active themselves. Be a good role model.

THE ULTIMATE HEALTHY EATING PLAN

Increase the amount of time and energy you spend in activities of daily living (take the stairs, not the elevator). Enjoy a minimum of 30 minutes, and ideally 45 minutes to 1 hour, of planned, moderate-intensity physical activity on most and preferably all days of the week. Brisk walking and resistance exercises (lifting weights) are highly recommended activities.

RESEARCH HIGHLIGHT

Dieting by cutting back on calories may decrease your body's ability to burn fat once you stop dieting. In a Netherlands study, however, men who combined regular physical activity with a lower calorie diet were able to counteract this decline. Research shows that a calorie-restricted diet combined with both aerobic exercise (like jogging, cycling or brisk walking) and resistance strength training (working out with weights) is optimal for helping you lose body fat while preserving and building lean muscle tissue.

RESEARCH HIGHLIGHT

In a study from Johns Hopkins University, resistance training or working out with weights boosted metabolism (calorie-burning) for 2 hours after working out, while the increase in calorie burning from aerobic exercise like jogging lasted for less than an hour afterward. A good exercise plan includes both aerobic exercise and resistance training exercise.

Putting It
All Together

Now that you understand the key elements that make up the Ultimate Healthy Eating Plan, it's time to get started. Here are some important tips to keep in mind on your way.

Top Seven "Getting Started" Tips

1 Before starting any new eating plan or exercise program, be sure to check with your family doctor. It's also a great idea to get your blood pressure, blood cholesterol and weight checked at this time so you can see what a difference the Plan makes for you (see page 276–277 for healthy weight, blood pressure and blood cholesterol levels).

2 Take it slow, one step at a time. Don't feel you have to adopt every single aspect of the Plan overnight. You may want to start by adding more vegetables, fruit and whole grains to your diet and then slowly introduce other foods like flax and beans. This slow progress is especially important if your current diet falls into the less-than-healthy category. It takes times for your body to adjust to all these healthy foods, including the higher amounts of fiber.

3 Don't forget your water. Because the Plan is high in fiber, it's important to drink lots of water each day in order to keep things moving along (if you know what I mean).

4 If one of Mairlyn's recipes contains an ingredient you haven't used before (maybe mango chutney or kale), please don't shy away from trying it. Mairlyn has done her best to stick to ingredients that are now widely available at most supermarkets. She uses these ingredients because of the wonderful flavor, nutrition or disease-fighting potential they provide.

5 This plan can be used with children over the age of two, but much smaller serving sizes are recommended. For example, most preschoolers should consume only about one-quarter to one-half the suggested servings. Also remember the "age + 5" rule when determining how many grams of fiber your child should have each day. This means, for example, that you can give young children whole-grain cereals, but don't add extra fiber by topping the cereal off with All Bran or Bran Buds.

6 The suggested meal plans that follow are meant to act as guidelines only. Please feel free to adapt them to suit your needs, likes and dislikes. For example, although a different kind of whole-grain cereal is listed for most days of the week, you may choose to limit your selection to one or two different cereals most of the time. The same goes for vegetables and fruits. While variety in this category is important, you may choose to eat more strawberries one week because they're in season and on sale.

7 Be a planner. A huge (and I do mean huge!) part of being a healthy eater is to be willing to spend a small amount of time each week planning. This includes things like:

- planning your meals for the week (especially dinners) and making sure you have all the necessary ingredients on hand

- making a double batch of muffins on the weekend so you can enjoy them during the week

- always packing the recommended snacks like fruit or nuts in your briefcase, purse or knapsack before you leave home each day (you don't want to end up playing vending-machine roulette!)

- getting your lunch ready the night before and getting tomorrow night's dinner organized ahead of time

SUMMARY OF THE ULTIMATE HEALTHY EATING PLAN RECOMMENDATIONS

Use the following recommendations to guide your daily food choices.

ADDED FATS
3 TO 6 SERVINGS DAILY

ONE FAT SERVING

1 tsp (5 mL) extra virgin olive oil or canola oil

1 tsp (5 mL) nonhydrogenated margarine

1 tbsp (15 mL) light or low-fat mayonnaise

1 tbsp (15 mL) light or low-fat salad dressing

GOOD ADVICE

Choose products (margarine, salad dressing, mayonnaise and spreads) made primarily with either extra virgin olive oil or canola oil.

Buy light or low-fat salad dressings and mayonnaise that contain about 3 to 4 grams of fat per serving. Do not buy fat-free versions of these products.

Exceptions to the rule: Consume 1 less serving of added fats on the days you eat soy nuts. Consume 2 less servings of added fats on the days you eat a full serving (2 tbsp/25 mL) of peanut butter. Consume an extra serving of fat on the days you don't have nuts of any kind.

Count 8 large olives as 1 serving of fat, count 1/4 avocado as 2 servings of fat.

VEGETABLES AND FRUIT
5 TO 10 SERVINGS DAILY

ONE SERVING OF FRUIT OR VEGETABLES

1 medium-size vegetable or fruit

1/2 cup (125 mL) raw, cooked or frozen vegetable or fruit

1/2 cup (125 mL) vegetable or fruit juice

1 cup (250 mL) salad

1/4 cup (50 mL) dried fruit

GOOD ADVICE

At least half of your daily intake of vegetables and fruit should be dark green, orange or red in color.

Enjoy cruciferous vegetables like kale, broccoli, Brussels sprouts and cauliflower at least three times during the week and ideally more.

When possible, also make berries or dried fruits a regular part of your diet and regularly enjoy tomatoes and tomato-based foods.

Use the following recommendations to guide your daily food choices.

GRAINS
5 TO 12 SERVINGS OF GRAIN PRODUCTS DAILY

ONE SERVING OF GRAINS (most, and ideally all, should be whole grain)	1 slice whole-grain bread 1/2 whole-grain hamburger bun 1/2 whole-grain English muffin 1/2 whole-grain small bagel 1/2 of a 6-inch (15-cm) whole-grain pita bread 1 (6-inch/15-cm) whole-grain tortilla 1/2 cup (125 mL) brown rice 1/2 cup (125 mL) whole-wheat pasta 1/2 cup (125 mL) whole-wheat couscous 1 oz (30 g) whole-grain ready-to-eat cereal (that's about 3/4 to 1 cup/175 to 250 mL of most cereals; the cereal box label indicates what 1 oz/30 g represents) 3/4 cup (175 mL) whole-grain, cooked cereal 3 to 4 small whole-grain crackers 1 (4-inch/10-cm) whole-grain pancake 1 small whole-grain muffin
GOOD ADVICE	Enjoy whole-grain cereal for breakfast most days of the week. Minimize your intake of refined grains—no more than about 1 to 2 servings per day if at all.

MILK PRODUCTS
3 TO 4 LOWER FAT SERVINGS DAILY

ONE SERVING OF MILK PRODUCTS	1 cup (250 mL) milk 1 cup (250 mL) buttermilk 2 slices (2 oz or 50 g) cheese 3/4 cup (175 g) yogurt 4 tablespoons (60 mL) grated Parmesan cheese 1/2 cup (125 mL) ricotta cheese
ONE-HALF SERVING OF MILK PRODUCTS	3/4 cup (175 mL) ice cream 1/2 cup (125 mL) frozen yogurt 1 cup (250 mL) cottage cheese
GOOD ADVICE	For vitamin D, 2 of your 3 to 4 servings should be in the form of low-fat milk on most days of the week.

MEAT AND MEAT ALTERNATIVES
2 TO 3 SERVINGS OF MEAT OR MEAT ALTERNATIVES DAILY

MEAT ALTERNATIVES	fish eggs nuts and beans, including soy

Use the following recommendations to guide your daily food choices.

BEANS
3 TO 5 SERVINGS EACH WEEK

ONE SERVING OF BEANS	1/2 cup (125 mL) beans

SOY
1 TO 2 SERVINGS ON MOST DAYS OF THE WEEK

ONE SERVING OF SOY	1 cup (250 mL) fortified soy milk
	1/2 cup (125 mL) tofu
	3 tbsp (45 mL) soy nuts
	1 veggie burger (or other meat replacement product made with soy protein—look for those containing about 10 g of soy protein/serving)
GOOD ADVICE	One serving of fortified soy milk can be used as a replacement to 1 serving of cow's milk (when used in this way, count as a milk alternative not a meat alternative).

EGGS
NO MORE THAN 3 TO 4 TIMES PER WEEK

ONE SERVING	1 egg
GOOD ADVICE	Always choose omega-3 eggs.

MEAT
NO MORE THAN 1 SERVING DAILY

ONE SERVING OF MEAT	2 to 3 oz (60 to 85 g) lean meat or poultry
	2 slices of lean cold cuts (3-in x 3-in x 1/4-in / 7 1/2-cm x 7 1/2-cm x 1/2-cm)
GOOD ADVICE	Limit red meat to no more than twice a week.
	Choose chicken or turkey more often—always remove the skin.

FISH
2 SERVINGS OF HIGHER FAT FISH (LIKE SALMON, MACKEREL, HERRING, RAINBOW TROUT) EACH WEEK

ONE SERVING OF FISH	3 oz (85 g) of cooked fish (about the size of a deck of cards)
	3/4 cup (175 mL) flaked or canned fish

NUTS
1/2 TO 1 SERVING FIVE TIMES EACH WEEK

ONE SERVING OF NUTS	1 oz (30 g) of nuts—a small handful or about 1/4 cup (50 mL)
	2 tbsp (25 mL) peanut butter —about the size of a ping-pong ball

Use the following recommendations to guide your daily food choices.

FLAX
1 TO 2 SERVINGS DAILY

ONE SERVING	1 tbsp (15 mL) ground flaxseed

TEA
3 TO 6 CUPS OF GREEN OR BLACK TEA DAILY

ONE SERVING	a typical cup of tea is 3/4 cup/175 mL

WATER
(OR OTHER FLUIDS LIKE MILK OR JUICE): 6 TO 8 CUPS (1.5 TO 2 L) DAILY

GOOD ADVICE	Count every cup of tea as 1/2 cup (125 mL) of water.

ALCOHOL
(WINE, BEER, LIQUOR)

MODERATE	If you choose to drink, limit intake to no more than 2 drinks for men and 1 drink for women each day.

CHOCOLATE
NO MORE THAN 1 SMALL SERVING DAILY

Ideally, use chocolate to make healthy foods taste better. For example, add chocolate chips to whole-grain muffins, pancakes or trail mix.

Choose mostly chocolate that contains higher amounts of flavonoids, such as M&M's Chocolate Candies.

EXERCISE
EVERY DAY

Increase the amount of time and energy you spend in activities of daily living (take the stairs, not the elevator). Enjoy a minimum of 30 minutes, and ideally 45 minutes to 1 hour, of planned, moderate-intensity physical activity on most and preferably all days of the week.

Brisk walking and resistance exercises (lifting weights) are highly recommended activities.

Recommended Number of Servings Within Each Food Category

In certain food categories a range of recommended servings is provided. For example, the recommendation for grains is to consume between 5 and 12 servings daily. These ranges are provided to suit individual energy (calorie) needs. Generally, most women should consume the lower number of recommended servings within each food category (it's okay to go higher when it comes to vegetables and fruit). For most very active men—especially younger men—the higher number of recommended servings is more appropriate. Most other men can choose in between the lower and higher recommended number of servings.

OVERVIEW AND INTRODUCTION TO MEAL PLANS

There are four possible seven-day meal plans to help get you started on the Ultimate Healthy Eating Plan. Keep the following in mind:

- The Eating-on-the-Run Meal Plan is geared for super-quick dinners and eating away from home.

- The Summertime Meal Plan takes into account the wide variety of fresh vegetables and fruit that are available in summer.

- The Wintertime Meal Plan is designed around heartier meals and a more limited selection of fresh produce.

- The Weight-Loss Meal Plan (1600 calories per day) allows people to achieve healthy, realistic weight-loss goals.

- All the meal plans contain about 15-20% of calories from protein, 25-30% of calories from fat, 55-60% of calories from carbohydrate and 25-35 grams of fiber (all within recommended guidelines for good health).

- With the exception of the Eating-on-the-Run Meal Plan, all the plans average less than 2000 mg of sodium per day (recommended intake is 2400 mg or less). The Eating-on-the-Run Meal Plan is slightly higher in sodium, averaging just over 2400 mg per day, which is still pretty incredible for life in the fast lane.

- In terms of calories (with the exception of the Weight-Loss Meal Plan) all the meal plans average about 1900 calories per day. This is an appropriate calorie level for weight maintenance for most women. Men may choose to add additional servings of some of the foods to reach a level of about 2200 calories each day. Suggested additions for most men include an extra 1/2 serving of nuts, 2 servings of grains and 1 serving of fat.

The Seven-Day Eating-on-the-Run Meal Plan

This plan is geared for super-quick dinners and for eating away from home.

- This plan contains 1900 calories per day (it's closer to 1800 if you omit the sugar allowed on your cereal and in your tea).

- This plan is designed around a more limited selection of fresh vegetables and fruits. You can, however, increase the scope of your choices during those times of the year when a wider variety of fresh produce is available.

- One of the most challenging aspects of the Eating-on-the-Run Meal Plan is keeping the sodium numbers down. Most fast foods and processed foods are very high in salt. Choose less processed foods when you can, and buy convenience products that contain less salt (ideally less than 500 mg of sodium per serving).

Day 1 | Sunday

Breakfast

1 egg (cook in nonstick frying pan sprayed with no-stick cooking spray)
2 slices whole-wheat toast
2 tsp (10 mL) nonhydrogenated margarine
1 sliced tomato
1/2 cup (125 mL) calcium-fortified orange juice
tea with milk and 1 tsp (5 mL) sugar

Morning Snack

1 serving Big Blue Berry Purple Smoothie (page 247)
1 tbsp (15 mL) ground flaxseed (mix into smoothie)
tea with milk and 1 tsp (5 mL) sugar

Lunch

salmon salad sandwich
2 slices whole-wheat bread
2 oz (60 g) drained, canned salmon
1 tbsp (15 mL) light mayonnaise
6 baby carrots
1 glass (1 cup/250 mL) skim milk
tea with milk and 1 tsp (5 mL) sugar

- This is a fast, easy way to add some salmon to a busy week.

- When it comes to salmon, tuna, chicken or turkey salad sandwiches, I suggest you make your own or get your sandwich made to order with small quantities of light mayo (no more than 1 to 2 tablespoons/15 to 25 mL max). Most food court or restaurant versions of these sandwiches contain regular mayonnaise and usually lots of it.

THE SEVEN-DAY EATING-ON-THE-RUN MEAL PLAN

MEAL	SUNDAY	MONDAY	TUESDAY
BREAKFAST	Egg, Whole-Wheat Toast, Orange Juice, Sliced Tomato, Tea	Shreddies, All Bran, Flax, Skim Milk, Orange Juice, Tea	Cheerios, Bran Buds, Flax, Skim Milk, Orange Juice, Tea

MORNING SNACK	Big Blue Berry Purple
	  Smoothie,
	Flax,
	Tea
		1/2 Whole-Wheat
		  Bagel,
		Tea
			Almonds,
			Kiwi,
			Tea

LUNCH	Salmon Salad
	Sandwich (light
	  mayo),
	Baby Carrots,
	Skim Milk,
	Tea
		Wendy's Restaurant:
		Small Chili,
		Milk,
		Tea,
		Baby Carrots
			Harvey's:
			Veggie Burger (light
			  mayo, lettuce,
			  tomatoes),
			Baby Carrots,
			Milk,
			Tea

AFTERNOON SNACK	McDonald's Small
	  Vanilla Cone
		Roasted Soy Nuts,
		Apple
			Dried Apricots,
			Chocolate-Covered
			  Raisins

DINNER	President's Choice
	  Italian Style Pasta &
	  Beans,
	Whole-Wheat Toast,
	Broccoli,
	Skim Milk
		Peanut Butter and
		  Banana Sandwich,
		Skim Milk
			Swiss Chalet:
			Quarter Chicken
			  (white meat),
			Baked Potato,
			Water

DESSERT OR EVENING SNACK	Apple,
	M&M's Mini Chocolate
	  Candies
		Mandarin Orange
		  Sections,
		Chocolate-Covered
		  Raisins
			Whole-Wheat Toast
			  and Honey,
			Skim Milk

WEDNESDAY	THURSDAY	FRIDAY	SATURDAY
Raisin Bran, Flax, Skim Milk, Orange Juice, Tea	Instant Oatmeal, Flax, Raisins, Skim Milk, Orange Juice, Tea	Cheerios, Bran Buds, Flax, Skim Milk, Orange Juice, Tea	Post Fruit & Fibre, Flax, Skim Milk, Orange Juice, Tea
Walnuts, Apple, Tea	Peanuts, Banana, Tea	Soy Nuts, Dried Apricots, Tea	Super Chocolate Banana Soy Shake, Tea
Subway: Roast Beef Submarine Sandwich (lettuce, tomato, light mayo), Skim Milk, Kiwi, Tea	Grilled Chicken Sandwich, (light mayo, lettuce, tomato), Skim Milk, Tea	Restaurant Salad Bar: (dark leafy greens, broccoli, carrots, chickpeas), Skim Milk, Tea	Marinated Bean Salad (ready-made), Whole-Wheat Toast, Baby Carrots, Tea
Roasted Soy Nuts, Baby Carrots	Whole-Wheat Crackers, Kiwi	Café Latte, Two-Bite Brownie	Skim Milk, Kiwi
French Toast, Skim Milk	Baked Beans in Tomato Sauce, Whole-Wheat Toast, Broccoli, Baby Carrots, Water	Pizza, Baby Carrots, Skim Milk	Fine Dining: Poached or Grilled Salmon, Sautéed Veggies, Wild Rice, Red Wine
Red Grapes, M&M's Mini Chocolate Candies	Chocolate Soy Milk (heated and served with marshmallows)	Red Wine, Popcorn and Peanuts	Chocolate Sundae (low-fat frozen yogurt)

- Easy ways to get more salmon (or other higher fat fish) into your diet at dinnertime include any one of the following frozen fish convenience meals. Most of them you just pop in the oven and then serve. Good choices are Highliner's Salmon Fillets in Light Dill Sauce, President's Choice Honey Mustard Marinated Atlantic Salmon Fillets, President's Choice Dill and Cognac Marinated Salmon Fillets, President's Choice Salmon Burgers, President's Choice Peppered Smokey Rainbow Trout, and Master's Choice Wild Pacific Salmon Burgers. Stay away from breaded, deep-fried fish.

Afternoon Snack

1 small vanilla cone from McDonald's

- McDonald's cones are made with ice milk and contain less than 4 grams fat per cone. (A premium, high-fat ice cream often contains more than 16 grams fat per serving.)

- Best lunch or dinner choices at McDonald's: Small Hamburger, Chicken McGrill (without added sauce), Garden Salad McWrap or Chicken Salad McWrap. The McWraps do, however, contain twice as much sodium (about 1000 mg per wrap) as the hamburger (about 600 mg) due to the high salt content of the ready-made salad dressings.

- Ideally, your beverage of choice at McDonald's should be milk. Many fast-food restaurants carry only 2% milk. This is not the ideal choice (skim or 1% is best), but 2% is still a good option once in a while and within an overall, low-fat healthy eating plan. Most important, stay away from regular—as opposed to diet—soft drinks. A large Coca-Cola at McDonald's

contains over 300 calories and 20 teaspoons sugar. Who needs it?

- Beware of big burgers! One Big Xtra from McDonald's contains over 600 calories, 34 grams fat (and that's without the cheese) and almost 1400 mg of sodium. Those are Xtras we don't need!

Dinner

1 serving of President's Choice Italian Style Pasta & Beans (have one-third of what the box makes)
1 slice whole-wheat toast
1 tsp (5 mL) margarine
1 cup (250 mL) steamed or microwaved broccoli
1 tbsp (15 mL) Light Cheez Whiz (melt in microwave, pour over broccoli)
1 glass (1 cup/250 mL) skim milk

- This President's Choice product comes in a box and is usually found in the rice section of the supermarket. It's as easy to make as Kraft dinner but provides a lot more nutrition (including some beans!). It's very tasty and kids like it, too.

- Yes, it's okay to put a little bit of Light Cheez Whiz on your broccoli (especially if it means you'll eat three times as much broccoli!). One tablespoon (15 mL) contains about 33 calories, 1.7 grams fat, 123 mg sodium and 70 mg calcium.

Here are some important rules for buying healthier frozen dinners or prepackaged convenience meals

1 Choose lower fat meals—no more than 3 grams fat for every 100 calories.
2 Choose lower sodium meals—ideally less than 500 mg per serving. In some, the seasoning mix is packaged separately from the main meal; to reduce sodium, don't add all the seasoning mix.

3 When possible, choose meals that are higher in fiber—a minimum of 2 grams of fiber per serving and ideally 6 grams or more.

4 Supplement most convenience meals with veggies or whole grains from home.

Dessert or Evening Snack

1 apple

1/2 M&M's Mini Chocolate Candies tube (30-g tube)

- That's about 50 mini M&M's (if you're counting); if you have the regular size M&M's Chocolate Candies, limit yourself to about 20.

Day 2 | Monday

Breakfast

2/3 cup (150 mL) Shreddies cereal

1/4 cup (50 mL) All-Bran Buds cereal

1 tbsp (15 mL) ground flaxseed

2 tsp (10 mL) sugar to put on cereal (optional)

1 cup (250 mL) skim milk for cereal

1/2 cup (125 mL) calcium-fortified orange juice

tea with milk and 1 tsp (5 mL) sugar

- No matter how busy your day, always make time for cereal!

- If you're traveling, most hotels offer a high-fiber cereal like Raisin Bran on their menu. Order it!

Morning Snack

Tim Horton's Restaurant

1/2 whole-wheat bagel

1 tsp (5 mL) nonhydrogenated margarine

tea with milk and 1 tsp (5 mL) sugar

- Beware of bagels. Because of their size, most bagels are equal to at least three slices of bread

and contain 300 calories or more. That's why the Plan generally recommends just one-half bagel at each meal or at snack-time. Share the other half with a friend or save it for another meal.

- Stay away from donuts. They're deep-fried in those nasty hydrogenated fats.

- Beware of most commercially made muffins. Most contain between 300 and 400 calories and 20 grams fat or more. Low-fat muffins, while a better choice, still usually contain about 300 calories and few are made with 100% whole grains. Even if you're really busy, try to find time to make a big batch of one of our muffin recipes. Just freeze them and grab one when needed. They taste great, and they're probably the healthiest muffins you'll ever eat!

Lunch

Wendy's Restaurant

1 small Chili

1 carton of milk (1 cup/250 mL)

tea with milk and 1 tsp/5 mL sugar

6 baby carrots (packed in your bag)

- Even with a busy lifestyle, it's important to keep some healthy snacks in your purse, knapsack or briefcase. It's a great way to add more nutrition to your day, and it stops you from reaching for less-than-healthy snacks on the run.

- Other suggestions for lunch or dinner at Wendy's: Grilled Chicken Sandwich, Fresh Stuffed Pitas (with reduced-fat dressing on the side), Caesar Side Salad or Grilled Chicken Salad (reduced-fat dressing on the side), Garden Salad Bar (reduced-fat dressing on the side). When it comes to salad dressings, always go for light or low-fat options and limit yourself to 1 to 2 tablespoons (15 to 25 mL) max.

- If you like baked potatoes, keep in mind that one large potato at Wendy's rings in at over 300 calories. This is almost a meal in itself. So either make it a meal or share it with a friend (even a few friends). Stay away from those topped with cheese. The cheese adds anywhere from 14 to almost 24 grams of fat and 125 to 225 calories. Your best topping is 1 teaspoon (5 mL) of margarine. A small dollop of sour cream is also okay.

Afternoon Snack

3 tbsp (45 mL) roasted soy nuts

1 apple

- Make it a habit to drink water with most meals and snacks.

Dinner

peanut butter sandwich

2 slices whole-wheat bread

2 tbsp (25 mL) peanut butter

1 banana (slice and add to sandwich)

1 glass (1 cup/250 mL) skim milk

- A great dinner for life in the fast lane is simply a sandwich. It's fast, easy and, in most cases, a much better choice than a visit to your local fast-food restaurant. Cereal falls into the same category.

- A peanut butter sandwich is also a great dinner for kids—especially because so many kids can't bring peanut butter for lunch any more due to nut allergies.

Dessert or Evening Snack

16 chocolate-covered raisins

1/2 cup (125 mL) drained, canned mandarin orange sections

- Of all the types of canned fruit, I think mandarin orange sections are one of the tastiest. To reduce the calories and sugar, discard the syrup the fruit sits in.

Day 3 | Tuesday

Breakfast

1 cup (250 mL) Cheerios cereal

3 tbsp (45 mL) All-Bran Buds cereal

1 tbsp (15 mL) ground flaxseed

2 tsp (10 mL) sugar to put on cereal (optional)

1 cup (250 mL) skim milk for cereal

1/2 cup (125 mL) calcium-fortified orange juice

tea with milk and 1 tsp (5 mL) sugar

Morning Snack

12 almonds

1 kiwi

tea with milk and 1 tsp (5 mL) sugar

Lunch

Harvey's Restaurant

1 Veggie Burger (light mayo, extra lettuce and tomatoes)

1 milk (1 cup/250 mL)

tea with milk and 1 tsp (5 mL) sugar

6 baby carrots (packed in your bag—yes, you take them with you everywhere)

- Other suggestions for lunch or dinner at Harvey's: Grilled Chicken Sandwich and Garden Salad (reduced-fat dressing on the side).

- Waistline overload! One order of Poutine (fries, gravy and cheese—how's that for a combination?) contains over 700 calories and 40 grams fat. That's a meal your waistline doesn't need!

Afternoon Snack

1/4 cup (50 mL) dried apricots
16 chocolate-covered raisins

Dinner

Swiss Chalet Restaurant

1/4 chicken, white meat, skin removed
1/2 serving Chalet sauce
1/2 baked potato
1 tsp (5 mL) nonhydrogenated margarine
water

- Don't forget to take the skin off the chicken. A quarter chicken (white meat) with the skin contains 22 grams fat and 381 calories. The same meat with the skin removed contains 8 grams fat and 225 calories. Not to mention the fact that the skin contains mostly unhealthy-for-your-heart saturated fat.

- The Chalet Sauce (used for dipping your chicken into) is very low in fat and calories (24 calories, 0.5 grams fat per serving), but it's loaded with salt (570 mg of sodium). Use about half of the serving they give you.

- Other suggestions for lunch or dinner at Swiss Chalet: Grilled Chicken Salad (reduced-fat dressing on the side), Caesar Side Salad (reduced-fat dressing on the side), Chicken on a Kaiser (request white meat).

- Just say no! One large order of BBQ Back Ribs at Swiss Chalet contains over 800 calories and 50 grams fat. Now that's a heart attack on a plate!

- Another fast and healthy take-out meal is a rotisserie chicken from your local supermarket. Just don't forget to ditch the skin!

Dessert or Evening Snack

1 glass (1 cup/250 mL) skim milk
1 slice whole-wheat toast
1 tsp (5 mL) nonhydrogenated margarine
1 tsp (5 mL) honey

- A piece of whole-wheat toast with a bit of honey or jam is a healthy way to satisfy a craving for something sweet.

Day 4 | Wednesday

Breakfast

1 cup (250 mL) Raisin Bran cereal
1 tbsp (15 mL) ground flaxseed
2 tsp (10 mL) sugar to put on cereal (optional)
1 cup (250 mL) skim milk for cereal
1/2 cup (125 mL) calcium-fortified orange juice
tea with milk and 1 tsp (5 mL) sugar

Morning Snack

7 walnut halves
apple
tea with milk and 1 tsp (5 mL) sugar

Lunch

Take-out: Subway Restaurant

1 small Roast Beef Submarine Sandwich (made with Harvest Wheat Bread)
2 tbsp (30 mL) light or low-fat mayo (no pickles, no olives, made with extra lettuce and tomatoes)
1 carton (1 cup/250 mL) of skim milk
1 kiwi
tea with milk and 1 tsp (5 mL) sugar

Day 4 | Wednesday

Some important rules for healthy sub sandwiches

1 Always choose whole-grain buns (most are actually a mix of white flour and whole-wheat flour, but they're still a better choice than just white bread).

2 To limit sodium, hold the cheese, olives and pickles.

3 To limit fat, ask for light or low-fat mayo and either ask for it on the side or tell them exactly how much you want.

4 Go for veggies. Ask for extra lettuce and tomato slices.

5 To limit calories, choose small subs.

6 Although all subs are high in salt, the lowest-fat subs include lean ham, roast beef, chicken or turkey breast, and veggie subs.

7 Don't be a meathead! A typical meatball sub sandwich contains over 500 calories, 30 grams fat and a whopping 2000 mg sodium.

Afternoon Snack

3 tbsp (45 mL) roasted soy nuts
6 baby carrots

Dinner

1 serving French Toast (page 260)
3 tbsp (45 mL) light syrup or 4 tsp (20 mL) real maple syrup
1 tsp (5 mL) nonhydrogenated margarine
1 glass (1 cup/250 mL) skim milk

• French toast and pancakes are great for delicious dinners in a hurry. They're also a healthy way to satisfy cravings for something sweet.

Dessert or Evening Snack

1 cup (250 mL) red grapes
1/2 M&M's Mini Chocolate Candies tube (30-g tube)

• That's about 50 mini M&M's (if you're counting); if you have the regular size M&M's Chocolate Candies, limit yourself to about 20.

Day 5 | Thursday

Breakfast

1 packet instant oatmeal cereal with raisins
1 tbsp (15 mL) ground flaxseed
3/4 cup (175 mL) skim milk for cereal
1/2 cup (125 mL) calcium-fortified orange juice
tea with milk and 1 tsp (5 mL) sugar

Morning Snack

16 peanuts
1 banana
tea with milk and 1 tsp (5 mL) sugar

Lunch

Restaurant or cafeteria

grilled chicken breast sandwich (request whole-grain bun if available)
1 tbsp (15 mL) light mayonnaise
extra lettuce and tomatoes (no pickles)
1 carton (1 cup/250 mL) skim milk
tea with milk and 1 tsp (5 mL) sugar
6 baby carrots (packed in your bag)

• Research shows that people who regularly dine away from home consume more fat, more sodium and less vegetables and fruit. If you dine out a lot, be conscious of your choices.

Afternoon Snack

4 whole-wheat crackers
1 kiwi

• Few crackers are actually whole grain. Most are made either with white flour or a combination of white and whole-wheat flour. Triscuits are one of the few crackers that are whole grain. Choose the sodium-reduced variety.

Dinner

1 cup (250 mL) Heinz Beans in Tomato Sauce (warmed in microwave)

1 slice whole-wheat toast

1 tsp (5 mL) nonhydrogenated margarine

1 cup (250 mL) microwaved broccoli

1 tbsp (15 mL) Light Cheez Whiz (melted in microwave)

6 baby carrots

water

- Always keep a few cans of beans in your cupboards. They're great for super quick dinners and most kids love them, too. If you want to jazz them up a bit, try the Jazzy Bean recipe on page 242.

- Always keep your fridge stocked with frozen vegetables like broccoli, peas and corn. That way there's no excuse for not having veggies at dinnertime. The microwave is the fastest and easiest way to cook frozen veggies. It helps preserve the most nutrients as well.

Dessert or Evening Snack

1 cup (250 mL) chocolate-flavored soy milk

- Tasty option: Warm the soy milk in the microwave and top it off with a few mini-marshmallows.

Day 6 | Friday

Breakfast

1 cup (250 mL) Cheerios cereal

3 tbsp (45 mL) All-Bran Buds cereal

1 tbsp (15 mL) ground flaxseed

2 tsp (10 mL) sugar to put on cereal (optional)

1 cup (250 mL) skim milk for cereal

1/2 cup (125 mL) calcium-fortified orange juice

tea with milk and 1 tsp (5 mL) sugar

Morning Snack

3 tbsp (45 mL) roasted soy nuts

1/4 cup (50 mL) dried apricots

tea with milk and 1 tsp (5 mL) sugar

Lunch

Cafeteria or restaurant salad bar

2 cups (500 mL) dark leafy greens

1 cup (250 mL) raw veggies (broccoli, red peppers, carrots)

2 tbsp (25 mL) low-fat or light salad dressing

1/2 cup (125 mL) chickpeas or marinated bean salad

water

tea with milk and 1 tsp (5 mL) sugar

- When it comes to salad bars, steer clear of pre-mixed macaroni, potato or coleslaw salads. Most are loaded with fat. And remember that cheese—especially if it's not fat-reduced—is best consumed in small quantities.

Afternoon Snack

Second Cup Restaurant

1 regular size latte made with 1% milk

1 tsp (5 mL) sugar

1 Two-Bite Brownie (packed in your bag) OR split one of the treats on the menu with about four friends!

- Skip the specialty coffees with added syrups and whipped cream. The Crème Brulée Ristretto

Day 6 | Friday

with whipped cream, for example, contains 750 calories and 18 grams of fat. That's not a coffee. That's a meal and a half!

- Two-Bite Brownies are available at most supermarkets. They can be substituted for an alternative chocolate treat as listed in the "Leaving Room for Chocolate" chapter.

Dinner

Take-out pizza

2 slices thin-crust, vegetarian pizza
1 glass (1 cup/250 mL) skim milk

Here are some important rules for healthy pizza eating

1 Never eat more than two slices of a medium-size pizza. If you're still hungry, fill up on other foods like baby carrots or a salad with a low-fat or light dressing.
2 Go for a thin-crust pizza and ask for one-third to one-half the cheese. (I promise the pizza still tastes great and you won't notice the difference.)
3 Avoid topping your pizza with fatty meats like pepperoni, sausage and ground beef.
4 Always top your pizza with lots of fresh veggies. You can even ask for extra tomato sauce.

- Artery alert! Two slices of a medium Meat Lover's Stuffed Crust Pizza from Pizza Hut contains 1086 calories, 58 grams fat, and 2854 mg sodium!

- If you buy frozen pizza, look for the lower fat, thin-crust varieties. For example, one-quarter of a Del Maestro's thin crust, Vegetarian Pizza rings in at only 215 calories and 8.3 grams fat. President's Choice thin crust, Wood-burning Pizzas are also good.

Dessert or Evening Snack

It's Friday. Rent a movie and enjoy . . .

1 glass (5 oz/145 mL) red wine
3 cups (750 mL) light microwave popcorn
16 peanuts

Day 7 | Saturday

Breakfast

1 cup (250 mL) Post Fruit & Fibre cereal
1 tbsp (15 mL) ground flaxseed
2 tsp (10 mL) sugar to put on cereal (optional)
1 cup (250 mL) skim milk for cereal
1/2 cup (125 mL) calcium-fortified orange juice
tea with milk and 1 tsp (5 mL) sugar

Morning Snack

1 serving Super Chocolate Banana Soy Shake (page 245)
tea with milk and 1 tsp (5 mL) sugar

Lunch

1/2 cup (125 mL) ready-made bean salad
2 slices whole-wheat toast
2 tsp (10 mL) nonhydrogenated margarine
6 baby carrots
tea with milk and 1 tsp (5 mL) sugar

- If you're looking for a tasty, ready-made bean salad, try President's Choice Tex-Mex Bean and Corn Salad. Another good option is Unico's Insalata Toscana Marinated Bean Salad. Both these bean salads are found in the canned bean section of the supermarket. They are a super fast and easy way to enjoy more beans. They also pack well for brown bag lunches.

Afternoon Snack

1 kiwi

1 glass (1 cup/250 mL) skim milk

Dinner

Nice dinner on the town

5 oz (140 g) poached or grilled salmon

1 cup (250 mL) sautéed veggies

1 cup (250 mL) wild or brown rice

1 glass (5 oz/145 mL) red wine (go for an extra walk today to earn your glass of wine)

- Most restaurants serve much larger portion sizes than you need. It's not uncommon to get more than 9 oz (250 g) of fish or meat in one meal. This is a good time for a doggie bag!

- Sharing is a good word when it comes to restaurant meals. My husband and I often share an appetizer, share a light main course and then, if we really feel like indulging, share a little dessert. Whenever possible, we always follow up our meal with a good long walk.

Other recommended healthy appetizers or entrées

1 soups like minestrone loaded with veggies and beans

2 dark green leafy salads (ask for dressing on the side)

3 small filet mignon or sirloin steak

4 fajitas (go easy on the guacamole and sour cream)

5 stir-fries with lots of veggies and lean meats

6 chicken or turkey breast (not breaded and fried or smothered in a rich cream sauce)

7 tomato-based pasta dish

8 olive-oil based pasta dish (small serving to limit calories)

9 kebobs made with lean meat or chicken

Dessert

At home

1/2 cup (125 mL) low-fat, vanilla frozen yogurt

2 tsp (10 mL) chocolate syrup

- Most ready-made chocolate syrups (the kind you use to make chocolate milk) contain just a trace of fat (0.1 g) and about 36 calories per 2 teaspoon (10 mL) serving. They make low-fat vanilla frozen yogurt so much more fun to eat. For kids, add sprinkles on top!

THE SEVEN-DAY SUMMERTIME MEAL PLAN

MEAL	SUNDAY	MONDAY	TUESDAY
BREAKFAST	Whole-Wheat Blueberry Buttermilk Pancakes, Orange Juice, Tea	Shreddies, All-Bran, Skim Milk, Orange Juice, Blueberries, Tea	Raisin Bran, Skim Milk, Orange Juice, Tea
MORNING SNACK	Low-Fat Fruit-Flavored Yogurt, Tea	Banana Chocolate Chip Muffin, Plums, Tea	Banana Chocolate Chip Muffin, Apricots, Tea
LUNCH	Summer Fiesta Chickpea Salad, Whole-Wheat Toast, Skim Milk, Tea	Peanut Butter & Banana Sandwich, Skim Milk, Tea	Brown Rice Risotto with Kale & Squash (leftover from Sunday), 1/2 Whole-Wheat Bagel, Skim Milk, Tea
AFTERNOON SNACK	Super Chocolate Banana Soy Shake, Flax	Nectarine, Low-Fat Cheese	Walnuts, Kiwi
DINNER	Brown Rice Risotto with Kale & Squash, Green Salad (raspberry dressing), Skim Milk	Salmon with Mango Salsa, Broccoli, Brown Rice, Tomato Juice	Lemon Chicken, Corn on the Cob, Green Beans, Cherry Tomatoes, Skim Milk
DESSERT OR EVENING SNACK	Almonds, Kiwi	Chocolate Soy Milk	Super Soy Raspberry Smoothie

WEDNESDAY	THURSDAY	FRIDAY	SATURDAY
Cheerios, Bran Buds, Skim Milk, Orange Juice, Flax, Strawberries, Tea	Instant Oatmeal, Raisins, Flax, Skim Milk, Orange Juice, Tea	Shreddies, All-Bran, Skim Milk, Orange Juice, Strawberries, Tea	Post Fruit & Fibre, Orange Juice, Flax, Blueberries, Tea
Chocolate or Coffee-Flavored Soy Milk	Roasted Soy Nuts, Apricots, Tea	Banana Chocolate Chip Muffin, Nectarine, Tea	Whole-Wheat Toast & Jam, Tea
Tuna Salad Sandwich (light mayo, red peppers), Baby Carrots, Skim Milk, Tea	Turkey Sandwich (light mayo, lettuce, tomatoes), Green Salad (raspberry dressing), Skim Milk	Hummus with Roasted Red Peppers, Whole-Wheat Pita Bread, Baby Carrots, Skim Milk, Tea	Strawberry & Spinach Salad with Almonds, Whole-Wheat Toast, Skim Milk, Tea
Gorp (trail mix with nuts, dried fruit & chocolate chips)	Two-Bite Brownie, Apple, Tea	Roasted Soy Nuts, Tomato Juice	Roasted Soy Nuts
Beef Kebobs, Brown Rice, Green Salad (house dressing), Homemade Iced Tea	Amazing Black Bean Quesadillas, Skim Milk	Baked Salmon with Fresh Citrus, Roasted Garlic Potatoes, Asparagus with Balsamic Vinegar, Skim Milk	Chicken with Mango & Apricots, Brown Rice, Broccoli, Red Wine
Cantaloupe (drizzled with honey and lime juice)	Watermelon	Popcorn, Red Wine	Strawberries with French Vanilla Yogurt

The Seven-Day Summertime Meal Plan

The Summertime Meal Plan takes into account the wide variety of fresh vegetables and fruit that are available in summer.

- This plan contains 1900 calories per day (closer to 1800 calories if you omit the sugar allowed on your cereal and in your tea).

- Start by reviewing all seven days and prepare your grocery list based on the suggested recipes.

- Don't forget, if you're having a really busy day you can substitute one of the recommended convenience meals from the Seven-Day Eating-on-the-Run Meal Plan.

Day 1 | Sunday

Breakfast

1 serving Whole-Wheat Blueberry Buttermilk Pancakes (page 259)
1 tsp (5 mL) nonhydrogenated margarine
3 tbsp (45 mL) light syrup OR 4 tsp (20 mL) maple syrup
1/2 cup (125 mL) calcium-fortified orange juice
tea with milk and 1 tsp (5 ml) sugar

- Real maple syrup is delicious, but it's also a concentrated source of calories at 52 calories per tablespoon (15 mL). That means you should either use it in small quantities or try one of the "light" syrups. They contain half the calories and still have very good flavor.

- The Plan averages 3 servings of milk products daily, but I still recommend calcium-fortified orange juice to ensure calcium needs are met. This is especially important for teenagers and the over-50 crowd, as calcium requirements are significantly higher during these times. In terms of taste, I say Tropicana can't be beat.

Morning Snack

1 small container (175 g) low-fat, fruit-flavored yogurt
tea with milk and 1 tsp (5 mL) sugar

- Check the yogurt label and look for brands that contain added acidophilus, casei or bifidus cultures. These bacteria may actually be good for your health.

Lunch

1 serving Summer Fiesta Chickpea Salad (page 228)
1 slice of whole-wheat toast
1 tsp (5 mL) nonhydrogenated margarine
1 glass (1 cup/250 mL) skim milk
tea with milk and 1 tsp (5 mL) sugar

- This salad can be made the day before. It keeps well in the fridge for up to one week.

Afternoon Snack

1 Super Chocolate Banana Soy Shake (page 245)
1 tbsp (15 mL) ground flaxseed (stir into shake)

- While the type of fat found in soy milk is not the same as the unhealthy-for-your-heart saturated kind found in milk products, it's still a good idea to choose lower fat brands to limit your calorie intake. This choice leaves room in your diet for the fats we recommend, including extra virgin olive oil, canola oil, flaxseed, fish and nuts.

Dinner

1 serving Short-Grain Brown Rice Risotto with Kale and Squash (page 181)
2 cups (500 mL) dark leafy green salad with 2 tbsp (25 mL) Unbelievably Delicious Raspberry Salad Dressing (page 146)
1 glass (1 cup/250 mL) skim milk

- Because this risotto takes a little bit more time to cook it's ideal for making on the weekend. If you haven't tried kale before, you'll find that this is a super tasty way to enjoy it for the first time.

Dessert or Evening Snack

12 almonds
1 kiwi

- If you think that eating a mere 12 almonds (1/2 serving nuts) seems barely worth the effort, think again. Most people find that nuts, even in small quantities, leave them feeling quite full.

Day 2 | Monday

Breakfast

2/3 cup (150 mL) Shreddies cereal
1/4 cup (50 mL) All-Bran Buds cereal
1/2 cup (125 mL) blueberries
2 tsp (10 mL) sugar to put on cereal (optional)
1 cup (250 mL) skim milk for cereal
1/2 cup (125 mL) calcium-fortified orange juice
tea with milk and 1 tsp (5 mL) sugar

- This meal plan allows you to add sugar to your tea and to your cereal. When consumed in moderation as part of a healthy diet, sugar is not associated with disease. If you wish to omit the sugar from the meal plan or use a sugar substitute, you will save yourself almost 100 calories each day.

Morning Snack

1 Banana Chocolate Chip Muffin (page 253)
tea with milk and 1 tsp (5 mL) sugar
2 plums

Day 2 | Monday

Lunch

peanut butter sandwich
2 slices whole-wheat bread
2 tbsp (25 mL) peanut butter
1 banana (slice and add to sandwich)
1 glass (1 cup/250 mL) skim milk
tea with milk and 1 tsp (5 mL) sugar

- Make it a habit to also drink water with most meals and snacks.

Afternoon Snack

1 nectarine
2 oz (60 g) low-fat cheese

Dinner

1 serving of Salmon with Mango Salsa (page 217)
1/2 cup (125 mL) steamed or microwaved broccoli
1/2 cup (125 mL) brown rice
1 tsp (5 mL) nonhydrogenated margarine (for broccoli or brown rice)
1/2 cup (125 mL) tomato juice

- To save time, make the salsa the night before.

- Don't forget to make twice as much brown rice as you need. That way you'll have enough for Wednesday night's dinner. Simply reheat it in the microwave with a little water and serve.

Dessert or Evening Snack

1 glass (1 cup/250 mL) chocolate soy milk

- Even though it's summertime, I still recommend warming your soy milk in the microwave and topping it with a few mini-marshmallows. Delicious!

Day 3 | Tuesday

Breakfast

1 cup (250 mL) Raisin Bran cereal
2 tsp (10 mL) sugar to put on cereal (optional)
1 cup (250 mL) skim milk for cereal
1/2 cup (125 mL) calcium-fortified orange juice
tea with milk and 1 tsp (5 mL) sugar

Morning Snack

1 Banana Chocolate Chip Muffin (page 253)
tea with milk and 1 tsp (5 mL) sugar
2 apricots

Lunch

1 serving Short-Grain Brown Rice Risotto with Kale and Squash (leftover from dinner on Sunday night)
1 glass (1 cup/250 mL) skim milk
1/2 whole-wheat bagel
1 tsp (5 mL) nonhydrogenated margarine
tea with milk and 1 tsp (5 mL) sugar

- Most bagels are equal to at least 3 slices of bread and contain 300 calories or more. That's why the Plan generally recommends enjoying just half a bagel at each meal or at snack-time. (Share the other half with a friend or save it for another meal.)

Afternoon Snack

7 walnut halves
1 kiwi

- A convenient way to eat a kiwi is simply to cut it in half and scoop it out with a spoon. Kids love to eat them this way!

Dinner

1 serving Lemon Chicken (page 206)

1/2 cup (125 mL) steamed or microwaved green
  beans

1 small cob of corn

1 1/2 tsp (7 mL) nonhydrogenated margarine (for
  beans and corn)

3 cherry tomatoes sliced in half, drizzled with 1/2
  tsp (2 mL) extra virgin olive oil

1 glass (1 cup/250 mL) skim milk

• To save time, marinate the chicken the night
  before.

Dessert or Evening Snack

1 Super Soy Raspberry Smoothie (page 247)

Day 4 | Wednesday

Breakfast

1 cup (250 mL) Cheerios cereal

3 tbsp (45 mL) All-Bran Buds cereal

1 tbsp (15 mL) ground flaxseed

1/2 cup (125 mL) strawberries

2 tsp (10 mL) sugar to put on cereal (optional)

1 cup (250 mL) skim milk for cereal

1/2 cup (125 mL) calcium-fortified orange juice

tea with milk and 1 tsp (5 mL) sugar

Morning Snack

1 cup (250 mL) of chocolate or coffee-flavored soy
  milk

• Give one of the new coffee-flavored soy milks
  like So Good Soyaccino a try. They have a rich
  flavor and come in small cartons.

Lunch

tuna salad sandwich

2 slices whole-wheat bread

2 oz (60 g) drained, canned white tuna

1 tbsp (15 mL) light mayonnaise

1/4 cup (50 mL) diced red pepper

6 baby carrots

1 glass (1 cup/250 mL) skim milk

tea with milk and 1 tsp (5 mL) sugar

• Make sure you buy white or albacore tuna to
  maximize your intake of healthy omega-3 fats.

Afternoon Snack

1 serving Gorp or trail mix (page 264)

• Who said healthy eating couldn't be fun?

Dinner

1 serving Beef Kebobs (page 226)

1 cup (250 mL) brown rice

2 cups (500 mL) dark leafy green salad with 2 tbsp
  (25 mL) House Dressing (page 145)

1 cup (250 mL) homemade iced tea

• To save time, marinate the meat the night before.

• Iced tea recipe: Pour 2 cups (500 mL) boiling
  water over 4 bags of black or green tea. Steep 3
  to 5 minutes. Remove tea bags. Add sugar if
  desired (about 4 to 6 teaspoons/20 to 30 mL).
  Add 2 cups (500 mL) cold water and chill.
  Serves 4.

• Try to limit your consumption of barbecued or
  grilled meat, poultry or fish to a maximum of
  three times per week. For healthier grilling,
  follow the tips outlined on page 61.

Dessert or Evening Snack

1/4 medium cantaloupe

• Tasty option: drizzle with juice of one lime and
  1 tsp (5 mL) honey.

Day 5 | Thursday

Breakfast

1 packet instant oatmeal cereal

1/4 cup (50 mL) raisins

1 tbsp (15 mL) ground flaxseed

3/4 cup (175 mL) skim milk for oatmeal (don't use water!)

1/2 cup (125 mL) calcium-fortified orange juice

tea with milk and 1 tsp (5 mL) sugar

Morning Snack

3 tbsp (45 mL) roasted soy nuts

tea with milk and 1 tsp (5 mL) sugar

2 apricots

Lunch

turkey sandwich

2 slices whole-wheat bread

2 oz (60 g) lean turkey

1 tbsp (15 mL) light mayonnaise

2 cups (500 mL) dark leafy green salad with 2 tbsp (25 mL) Unbelievably Delicious Raspberry Salad Dressing (page 146)

1 glass (1 cup/250 mL) skim milk

- Most processed luncheon meats are loaded with salt. Use either fresh meat (for example, cold leftover chicken or turkey from a previous dinner) or buy brands of processed meat that are lower in sodium. Schneider's Lifestyle line has over 30% less salt than regular luncheon meats.

- If you don't mind packing a sandwich to take for lunch each day but find it inconvenient to pack a salad, buy a side salad to go with your sandwich. Just be sure to choose dark leafy greens and ask for a light or low-fat salad dressing on the side (so you can control the quantity). The advantage of using one of our dressings is that they're all made with canola oil or extra virgin olive oil, they are much lower in sodium than most salad dressings, and perhaps most important, they taste great!

Afternoon Snack

1 Two-Bite Brownie (available at most supermarkets)

tea with milk and 1 tsp (5 mL) sugar

1 apple

- The brownie can be substituted for an alternative chocolate treat as listed in the Leaving Room for Chocolate chapter.

Dinner

1 serving Amazing Black Bean Quesadillas (page 234)

1 glass (1 cup/250 mL) skim milk

Dessert or Evening Snack

2 slices watermelon

Day 6 | Friday

Breakfast

2/3 cup (150 mL) Shreddies cereal

1/4 cup (50 mL) All-Bran Buds cereal

1/2 cup (125 mL) strawberries

2 tsp (10 mL) sugar to put on cereal (optional)

1 cup (250 mL) skim milk for cereal

1/2 cup (125 mL) calcium-fortified orange juice

tea with milk and 1 tsp (5 mL) sugar

Morning Snack

1 Banana Chocolate Chip Muffin (page 253)

tea with milk and 1 tsp (5 mL) sugar

1 nectarine

Lunch

hummus with pita bread

1 small (4-inch/10-cm) whole-wheat pita bread

1/4 cup (50 mL) Hummus with Roasted Red Peppers (page 229)

6 baby carrots

1 glass (1 cup/250 mL) skim milk

tea with milk and 1 tsp (5 mL) sugar

- If you don't have time to make hummus from scratch, buy it ready made. Look for lower fat brands. You can also mix a store-bought hummus with a bit of store-bought roasted red pepper dip—they go great together.

Afternoon Snack

3 tbsp (45 mL) roasted soy nuts

1/2 cup (125 mL) tomato juice

Dinner

1 serving Baked Salmon with Fresh Citrus (page 214)

1 serving Roasted Garlic Potatoes (page 177)

1 serving Asparagus with Balsamic Vinegar (page 172)

1 glass (1 cup/250 mL) skim milk

- This dinner sounds much more complicated than it is. Be sure to try it!

Dessert or Evening Snack

It's Friday, rent a movie and enjoy . . .

1 glass (5 oz/145 mL) red wine

3 cups (750 mL) light microwave popcorn

- Tasty option: Sprinkle popcorn with cinnamon and either a bit of icing sugar or a sugar substitute like Splenda.

Day 7 | Saturday

Breakfast

1 cup (250 mL) Post Fruit & Fibre cereal

3 tbsp (45 mL) All-Bran Buds cereal

1 tbsp (15 mL) ground flaxseed

1/2 cup (125 mL) blueberries

2 tsp (10 mL) sugar to put on cereal (optional)

1 cup (250 mL) skim milk for cereal

1/2 cup (125 mL) calcium-fortified orange juice

tea with milk and 1 tsp (5 mL) sugar

Morning Snack

1 slice whole-wheat toast with 1 tsp (5 mL) jam

tea with milk and 1 tsp (5 mL) sugar

Lunch

1 serving Strawberry and Spinach Salad with Almonds (page 148)

1 slice whole-wheat toast

1 tsp (5 mL) nonhydrogenated margarine

1 glass (1 cup/250 mL) skim milk

tea with milk and 1 tsp (5 mL) sugar

Afternoon Snack

3 tbsp (45 mL) roasted soy nuts

Dinner

1 serving Chicken with Mango and Apricots (page 198)

1 cup (250 mL) brown rice (pour some of the sauce from the chicken over the rice)

1/2 cup (125 mL) steamed or microwaved broccoli

1 glass (5 oz/145 mL) red wine

- This is a great dinner to serve for company!

- To earn your glass of wine, go for a walk after dinner.

Dessert or Evening Snack

1 serving Strawberries with French Vanilla Yogurt (page 248)

THE SEVEN-DAY WINTERTIME MEAL PLAN

MEAL	SUNDAY	MONDAY	TUESDAY
BREAKFAST	Apple & Oat Pancakes, Orange Juice, Tea	Mini-Wheats, All-Bran Buds, Skim Milk, Orange Juice, Banana, Tea	Shreddies, All-Bran Buds, Skim Milk, Orange Juice, Banana, Tea
MORNING SNACK	Ruby Red Grapefruit, Tea	Super Nutritious Chocolate Chip Bran Muffin, Tea	Super Nutritious Chocolate Chip Bran Muffin, Tea
LUNCH	Scrambled Eggs, Whole-Wheat Toast, Grape Tomato Salad, Skim Milk, Tea	Peanut Butter & Banana Sandwich, Skim Milk, Tea	Out-of-this-World Chili (leftover from Sunday), Green Salad (raspberry dressing), Skim Milk, Tea
AFTERNOON SNACK	Low-Fat Double Chocolate Fudge Pudding	Kiwi, Dried Apricots	Walnuts, Mandarin Orange
DINNER	Out-of-this-World Chili, Whole-Wheat Toast, Green Salad (house dressing), Skim Milk	Salmon Teriyaki, Broccoli & Red Pepper Stir-Fry, Brown Rice, Skim Milk	Sundried Tomato Pesto with Chicken & Rotini, Green Peas, Water
DESSERT OR EVENING SNACK	Dried Fruit Compote, Low-Fat Frozen Yogurt	Chocolate Soy Milk (heated & served with marshmallows)	Skim Milk, Chocolate-Covered Raisins

WEDNESDAY	THURSDAY	FRIDAY	SATURDAY
Raisin Bran, Flax, Skim Milk, Orange Juice, Banana, Tea	Cheerios, All-Bran Buds, Skim Milk, Orange Juice, Banana, Tea	Instant Oatmeal, Raisins, Skim Milk, Orange Juice, Tea	Cheerios, All-Bran Buds, Skim Milk, Orange Juice, Banana, Tea
Roasted Soy Nuts, Red Grapes	Super Nutritious Chocolate Chip Bran Muffin, Tea	Super Nutritious Chocolate Chip Bran Muffin, Tea	Whole-Wheat Toast & Jam, Tea
Tuna Salad Sandwich (light mayo), Skim Milk, Tea	Hummus with Roasted Red Peppers, Whole-Wheat Pita Bread, Sliced Tomato, Kiwi, Skim Milk, Tea	Green Salad (raspberry dressing), Walnuts, Whole-Wheat Roll, Skim Milk, Tea	Tex-Mex Bean & Corn Salad, Whole-Wheat Toast, Green Salad (house dressing), Skim Milk, Tea
Almonds, Baby Carrots	Peanuts, Dried Apricots	Roasted Soy Nuts, Mandarin Orange	Super Soy Strawberry Smoothie, Flax
Mairlyn's Amazing Tomato Sauce & Whole-Wheat Spaghetti, Green Salad (house dressing), Skim Milk	Poached Salmon with Mairlyn's World Famous Lime Mayo, Honey-Glazed Carrots, Broccoli, Orange Bulgar, Skim Milk	Marvelous Minestrone Soup, Whole-Wheat Toast, Skim Milk	Chicken Tarragon, Brown Rice, Stir-Fried Brussels Sprouts & Carrots, Red Wine
Pear, M&M's Mini Chocolate Candies	Super Chocolate Banana Soy Shake	Red Wine, Popcorn	Leave Room for . . . Chocolate Cake

The Wintertime Meal Plan is designed around heartier meals and a more limited selection of fresh produce.

- This plan contains 1900 calories per day (closer to 1800 calories if you omit the sugar allowed on your cereal and in your tea).

- Start by reviewing all seven days and prepare your grocery list based on the suggested recipes.

- Don't forget, if you're having a really busy day you can substitute one of the recommended convenience meals from the Seven-Day Eating-on-the-Run Meal Plan.

Day 1 | Sunday

Breakfast

1 serving Apple and Oat Pancakes (page 258)
1 tsp (5 mL) nonhydrogenated margarine
3 tbsp (45 mL) light syrup OR 4 tsp (20 mL) maple syrup
1/2 cup (125 mL) calcium-fortified orange juice
tea with milk and 1 tsp (5 mL) sugar

- These pancakes also make a great quick and easy dinner.

Morning Snack

1/2 ruby red grapefruit
1 tsp (5 mL) sugar (optional)
tea with milk and 1 tsp (5 mL) sugar

- Pink or red grapefruit is higher in beneficial plant compounds such as lycopene than white grapefruit.

Lunch

scrambled eggs (made with 1 whole egg and 1 egg white, use no-stick spray for cooking)
1 slice whole-wheat toast
1 tsp (5 mL) nonhydrogenated margarine
1 serving Grape Tomato Salad (page 152)
1 glass (1 cup/250 mL) skim milk
tea with milk and 1 tsp (5 mL) sugar

- By making scrambled eggs with 1 egg and 1 egg white (rather than 2 whole eggs), you keep your daily cholesterol intake within recommended guidelines.

Afternoon Snack

1 serving (1/2 cup/125 mL) ready made, low-fat chocolate pudding (such as Healthy Choice Double Chocolate Fudge Pudding)

- There are lots of ready-made, low-fat chocolate puddings available on grocery store shelves. They're good for chocolate cravings and help contribute to your daily calcium intake (most contain about 100 mg calcium per serving). For a treat, most kids love to dip chunks of fresh fruit into chocolate pudding.

Dinner

1 serving Out-of-this-World Chili (page 238)
1 slice whole-wheat toast
1 tsp (5 mL) nonhydrogenated margarine
2 cups (500 mL) dark leafy green salad with 2 tbsp (25 mL) House Dressing (page 145)
1 glass (1 cup/250 mL) skim milk

- This chili recipe is outstanding! It's also a great opportunity for you to try Yves Veggie Ground Round—a replacement for meat that's made out of soy. These types of products, which are now available in most supermarkets, make it just that much easier to get more soy into your diet.

Dessert or Evening Snack

1 serving Dried Fruit Compote (page 249)
1 small scoop (1/4 cup/50 mL) low-fat frozen yogurt

Day 2 | Monday

Breakfast

2/3 cup (150 mL) Mini-Wheats cereal
1/4 cup (50 mL) All-Bran Buds cereal
1/2 banana
1 cup (250 mL) skim milk for cereal
1/2 cup (125 mL) calcium-fortified orange juice
tea with milk and 1 tsp (5 mL) sugar

Morning Snack

1 Super Nutritious Chocolate Chip Bran Muffin (page 254)
tea with milk and 1 tsp (5 mL) sugar

Lunch

peanut butter sandwich
2 slices whole-wheat bread
2 tbsp (25 mL) peanut butter
1/2 banana (slice and add to sandwich)
1 glass (1 cup/250 mL) skim milk
tea with milk and 1 tsp (5 mL) sugar

- If you love chocolate milk (which, by the way, goes great with peanut butter sandwiches!), remember it's always better to make your own rather than buying the very rich, ready-made versions. Most ready-made chocolate milks, although low in fat, still contain an extra 70 calories or more per serving (1 cup/250 mL). When you make your own (add 1 tsp/5 mL chocolate syrup to a glass of skim milk) you are upping the calorie content only by about 18 calories.

Day 2 | Monday

- Yes, you can pack milk in your brown bag lunch and in your kids' lunch boxes! As soon as you wake up in the morning, simply pour milk—add a bit of chocolate syrup if you wish—into a Rubbermaid-type drinking box container (the kind with the straw). Put the container in the freezer while you're having your morning shower and eating your breakfast and then pop it in your lunch bag just before you head out the door. It will be cold and delicious and perfect for drinking at lunchtime!

Afternoon Snack

1 kiwi
1/4 cup (50 mL) dried apricots

- Make it a habit to drink water with most meals and snacks.

Dinner

1 serving Salmon Teriyaki (page 219)
1 serving Broccoli, Red Pepper and Fresh Ginger (page 173)
1/2 cup (125 mL) brown rice
1 tsp (5 mL) nonhydrogenated margarine
1 glass (1 cup/250 mL) skim milk

- If you don't have fresh salmon fillets on hand, you can use frozen. I always keep my freezer stocked with a box of President's Choice Atlantic Salmon fillets. They're fast, easy to defrost and taste great, too.

Dessert or Evening Snack

1 cup (250 mL) chocolate soy milk

- Tasty option: Warm the soy milk in the microwave and top it off with a few mini-marshmallows.

Day 3 | Tuesday

Breakfast

2/3 cup (150 mL) Shreddies cereal
1/4 cup (50 mL) All-Bran Buds cereal
1/2 banana
2 tsp (10 mL) sugar to put on cereal (optional)
1 cup (250 mL) skim milk for cereal
1/2 cup (125 mL) calcium-fortified orange juice
tea with milk and 1 tsp (5 mL) sugar

Morning Snack

1 Super Nutritious Chocolate Chip Bran Muffin (page 254)
tea with milk and 1 tsp (5 mL) sugar

Lunch

1 serving Out-of-this-World Chili (leftover from dinner on Sunday night)
2 cups (500 mL) dark leafy green salad with 2 tbsp (25 mL) Unbelievably Delicious Raspberry Salad Dressing (page 146)
1 glass (1 cup/250 mL) skim milk
tea with milk and 1 tsp (5 mL) sugar

- This salad dressing really is "unbelievably delicious!"

Afternoon Snack

7 walnut halves
1 mandarin orange

Dinner

1 serving Sundried Tomato Pesto with Chicken and Rotini (page 201)
1/2 cup (125 mL) steamed or microwaved green peas
1 tsp (5 mL) nonhydrogenated margarine
water

- Microwaving or steaming vegetables helps preserve most of the nutrients. If you boil vegetables, many of the water-soluble nutrients, like vitamin C, are lost in the water.

1 glass (1 cup/250 mL) skim milk
16 chocolate-covered raisins

- Don't forget—chocolate is best consumed and enjoyed in small quantities!

Day 4 | Wednesday
1 cup (250 mL) Raisin Bran cereal
1 tbsp (15 mL) ground flaxseed
2 tsp (10 mL) sugar to put on cereal (optional)
1 cup (250 mL) skim milk for cereal
1/2 cup (125 mL) calcium-fortified orange juice
tea with milk and 1 tsp (5 mL) sugar

3 tbsp (45 mL) roasted soy nuts
1/2 cup (125 mL) red grapes
tea with milk and 1 tsp (5 mL) sugar

tuna salad sandwich
2 slices whole-wheat bread
2 oz (60 g) drained, canned white tuna
1 tbsp (15 mL) light mayonnaise
1/4 cup (50 mL) diced red pepper
1 glass (1 cup/250 mL) skim milk
tea with milk and 1 tsp (5 mL) sugar

- Make sure you buy white or albacore tuna to maximize your intake of healthy omega-3 fats.

12 almonds
6 baby carrots

1 serving Mairlyn's Amazing Tomato Sauce (page 193)
1 1/2 cups (375 mL) whole-wheat pasta
2 cups (500 mL) dark leafy green salad with 2 tbsp (25 mL) House Dressing (page 145)
1 glass (1 cup/250 mL) skim milk

- If you don't have time to make spaghetti sauce from scratch (even though this recipe is super easy), buy ready-made sauces that are lower in sodium, such as the Healthy Choice line of sauces or the President's Choice Too-Good-To-Be-True line.

- Quote: "No man is lonely eating spaghetti; it requires so much attention."

1 pear
1/2 M&M's Mini Chocolate Candies tube (30-g tube)

- That's about 50 mini M&M's (if you're counting); if you have the regular size M&M's, limit yourself to about 20.

Day 5 | Thursday
1 cup (250 mL) Cheerios cereal
3 tbsp (45 mL) All-Bran Buds cereal
1/2 banana
2 tsp (10 mL) sugar to put on cereal (optional)
1 cup (250 mL) skim milk for cereal
1/2 cup (125 mL) calcium-fortified orange juice
tea with milk and 1 tsp (5 mL) sugar

Day 5 | Thursday

1 Super Nutritious Chocolate Chip Bran Muffin (page 254)

tea with milk and 1 tsp (5 mL) sugar

hummus with pita bread

1 small (4-inch/10cm) whole-wheat pita bread

1/4 cup (50 mL) Hummus with Roasted Red Peppers (page 229)

sliced tomato

1 kiwi

1 glass (1 cup/250 mL) skim milk

- If you don't have time to make hummus from scratch, buy ready-made hummus. Look for lower fat brands. You can also mix a store-bought hummus with a bit of store-bought roasted red pepper dip—they go great together.

16 peanuts

1/4 cup (50 mL) dried apricots

1 serving Poached Salmon with Mairlyn's World Famous Lime Mayo (page 218)

1 serving Honey Glazed Carrots (page 163)

1/2 cup (125 mL) steamed or microwaved broccoli (drizzle with lemon juice then top with a quick shake of light Parmesan cheese)

1 serving Orange Bulgar (page 183)

1 glass (1 cup/250 mL) skim milk

- Cooking salmon doesn't get any easier than this.

- If you've never had bulgar before, now's a great time to add a new whole grain to your repertoire.

1 serving Super Chocolate Soy Banana Shake (page 245)

Day 6 | Friday

1 packet instant oatmeal cereal

1/4 cup (50 mL) raisins

3/4 cup (175 mL) skim milk for oatmeal (don't use water!)

1/2 cup (125 mL) calcium-fortified orange juice

tea with milk and 1 tsp (5 mL) sugar

1 Super Nutritious Chocolate Chip Bran Muffin (page 254)

tea with milk and 1 tsp (5 mL) sugar

green salad with walnuts

2 cups (500 mL) dark leafy greens

2 tbsp (25 mL) Unbelievably Delicious Raspberry Salad Dressing (page 146)

7 walnut halves

1 whole-wheat roll

1 apple

1 glass (1 cup/250 mL) skim milk

tea with milk and 1 tsp (5 mL) sugar

3 tbsp (45 mL) roasted soy nuts

1 mandarin orange

1 serving Marvelous Minestrone Soup (page 156)

1 slice whole-wheat toast

1 tsp (5 mL) nonhydrogenated margarine

1 glass (1 cup/250 mL) skim milk

- Soup is a great vehicle for getting more beans into your diet. When you buy ready-made soups, look for lower sodium brands.

Dessert or Evening Snack

It's Friday, rent a movie and enjoy...

1 glass (5 oz/145 mL) of red wine

3 cups (750 mL) light microwave popcorn

- Tasty option: Sprinkle popcorn with a few shakes of light Parmesan cheese.

Day 7 | **Saturday**

Breakfast

1 cup (250 mL) Cheerios cereal

3 tbsp (45 mL) All-Bran Buds cereal

1/2 banana

2 tsp (10 mL) sugar to put on cereal (optional)

1 cup (250 mL) skim milk for cereal

1/2 cup (125 mL) calcium-fortified orange juice

tea with milk and 1 tsp (5 mL) sugar

Morning Snack

1 slice whole-wheat toast

1 tsp (5 mL) nonhydrogenated margarine

1 tsp (5 mL) jam

tea with milk and 1 tsp (5 mL) sugar

Lunch

1/2 cup (125 mL) ready-made bean salad

1 slice whole-wheat toast

1 tsp (5 mL) nonhydrogenated margarine

2 cups (500 mL) dark leafy green salad with 2 tbsp (25 mL) House Dressing (page 145)

1 glass (1 cup/250 mL) skim milk

tea with milk and 1 tsp (5 mL) sugar

- If you're looking for a tasty ready-made bean salad, try President's Choice Tex-Mex Bean and Corn Salad. Another option is Unico's Toscana Marinated Bean Salad. Both these bean salads are found in the canned bean section of the supermarket. They are a super fast and easy way to enjoy more beans. They also pack well for brown bag lunches.

Afternoon Snack

1 serving Super Soy Strawberrry Smoothie (page 247)

1 tbsp (15 mL) ground flaxseed (mix into smoothie)

Dinner

1 serving Chicken Tarragon (page 200)

1 serving Stir-Fried Brussels Sprouts and Carrots (page 175)

3/4 cup (175 mL) brown rice (pour some of the sauce from the chicken over rice)

1 glass (5 oz/145 mL) red wine

- This is a great dinner to serve to company!

Dessert or Evening Snack

1 serving Don't Forget to Leave Room for Chocolate Cake! (page 270)

- If you've exercised hard today, top the cake with chocolate icing. Otherwise, dust it with icing sugar.

THE SEVEN-DAY WEIGHT-LOSS MEAL PLAN

MEAL	SUNDAY	MONDAY	TUESDAY
BREAKFAST	French Toast, Orange Juice, Tea	Raisin Bran, Skim Milk, Orange Juice, Tea	Instant Oatmeal, Raisins, Flax, Skim Milk, Orange Juice, Tea
MORNING SNACK	Ruby Red Grapefruit, Tea	Pumpkin Chocolate Chip Muffin, Tea	Roasted Soy Nuts, Tea
LUNCH	Spinach & Egg Salad (house dressing), 1/2 Whole-Wheat Bagel, Skim Milk, Tea	Turkey Sandwich (light mayo, lettuce, tomato), Baby Carrots, Skim Milk, Tea	Mairlyn's World Famous Beans & Rice (leftover from Sunday), Whole-Wheat Roll, Skim Milk, Tea
AFTERNOON SNACK	Super Chocolate Banana Soy Shake, Flax	Peanuts, Cantaloupe	Almonds, Baby Carrots
DINNER	Mairlyn's World Famous Beans & Rice, Skim Milk	Salmon Chowder, Whole-Wheat Toast, Water	Chicken Burger, Green Salad (raspberry dressing), Water
DESSERT OR EVENING SNACK	Kiwi, Walnuts	Chocolate Soy Milk (warmed in microwave and served with mini marshmallows)	Skim Milk, M&M's Mini Chocolate Candies

WEDNESDAY	THURSDAY	FRIDAY	SATURDAY
Cheerios, All-Bran Buds, Skim Milk, Orange Juice, Tea	Shreddies, All-Bran Buds, Skim Milk, Orange Juice, Tea	Post Fruit & Fibre, Flax, Skim Milk, Orange Juice, Tea	Cheerios, All-Bran Buds, Skim Milk, Orange Juice, Tea

Pumpkin Chocolate
  Chip Muffin,
Tea
	Pumpkin Chocolate
	  Chip Muffin,
	Tea
		Roasted Soy Nuts,
		Tea
			Whole-Wheat Toast &
			  Jam,
			Ruby Red Grapefruit

Hummus with Roasted
  Red Peppers,
Whole-Wheat Pita,
Grape Tomato Salad,
Skim Milk,
Tea
	Tuna Salad Sandwich
	  (light mayo),
	Tea
		Spinach Salad with
		  Almonds (raspberry
		  dressing),
		Whole-Wheat Roll,
		Skim Milk
			Rotini with Plum
			  Tomatoes & Lentils
			  (leftover from
			  Friday),
			Skim Milk,
			Tea

Red Pepper Strips &
  Dip
	Skim Milk,
	Kiwi
		Two-Bite Brownie,
		Tea
			Super Soy Strawberry
			  Smoothie,
			Flax

Stir-Fried Broccoli with
  Cashews,
Brown Rice,
Skim Milk
	Salsa Baked Chicken,
	Brown Rice,
	Green Salad (house
	  dressing),
	Water
		Rotini with Plum
		  Tomatoes & Lentils,
		Baby Carrots,
		Skim Milk
			Company's Comin'
			  Salmon,
			Brussels Sprouts with
			  Maple Syrup,
			Wild & Brown Rice,
			Red Wine

Big Blue Berry Purple
  Smoothie
	Super Chocolate
	  Banana Soy Shake
		Red Wine,
		Popcorn
			Chocolate Fondue
			  with Fresh Fruit

The weight-loss plan at 1600 calories per day allows people to achieve healthy, realistic weight-loss goals.

- This plan is designed around a more limited selection of fresh vegetables and fruits. Be sure to increase the scope of your choices during those times of the year when a wider variety of fresh produce is available.

- Start by reviewing all seven days and prepare your grocery list based on the suggested recipes. (This is an essential step in any weight-loss plan!)

- This meal plan is designed around small meals (less than 500 calories per meal) and regular snacks. Research suggests that, especially as you age, you may not burn calories from fat as efficiently when you eat too many calories at one time. Eating regular meals and snacks also helps keep hunger at bay.

- Healthy weight loss is considered to be about 1 to 2 pounds (0.5 to 1 kg) or less per week.

- People with a healthy weight are less likely to develop diabetes, heart disease, stroke, gall-bladder disease, osteoarthritis and certain types of cancer such as colon cancer and post-menopausal breast cancer.

- Daily physical activity is essential to successful weight loss and the most important factor influencing weight maintenance. Make a weekly plan that summarizes how you will achieve your daily activity goals. Aim for a minimum of 45 minutes and ideally 1 hour of moderate-intensity activity each day. Walking is one of the best ways to get active! Be sure to review the Active Living for a Lifetime chapter.

- If you find it difficult to consume chocolate without overindulging, you may want to avoid chocolate entirely or limit chocolate treats to once a week.

- Minimum recommended daily food intake: 3 servings added fats, 5 servings vegetables and fruit, 5 servings whole grains, 2 servings milk, 1 serving fortified soy milk, 2 servings meat or alternatives (beans, nuts, fish, lean meat, eggs), 1 serving ground flax. Carry this list of recommended foods with you at all times. It will help you stay on course and allow you to keep track of what you need to eat each day.

Day 1 | **Sunday**

Breakfast

1 serving French Toast (page 260)

1 tsp (5 mL) nonhydrogenated margarine

2 tbsp (25 mL) light syrup OR 4 tsp (20 mL) maple syrup

1/2 cup (125 mL) calcium-fortified orange juice

tea with 1 tbsp/15 mL milk

Morning Snack

1/2 ruby red grapefruit

tea with 1 tbsp/15 mL milk

Lunch

spinach salad

2 cups (500 mL) spinach

2 tbsp (25 mL) House Dressing (page 145)

1 sliced hard-boiled egg

1/2 whole-wheat bagel

1 tsp (5 mL) margarine

1 glass (1 cup/250 mL) skim milk

tea with 1 tbsp/15 mL milk

- Drink water with most meals and snacks.

Afternoon Snack

1 serving Super Chocolate Banana Soy Shake (page 245)

1 tbsp (15 mL) ground flaxseed (mix into shake)

Dinner

1 serving Mairlyn's World Famous Beans and Rice (page 230)

1 glass (1 cup/250 mL) skim milk

- This is a delicious, bean-rich, fiber-rich meal. Research supports the fact that people who eat more fiber find it easier to lose weight and maintain a healthy weight.

Dessert or Evening Snack

1 kiwi

7 walnut halves

- If you think that eating a mere 7 walnut halves (1/2 serving nuts) seems like barely worth the effort, remember that most people find nuts, even in small quantities, leave them feeling quite full.

- Did you remember to exercise today? Physical activity during weight loss improves your metabolism (calorie-burning potential), your psychological well-being and your overall quality of life.

Day 2 | **Monday**

Breakfast

3/4 cup (175 mL) Raisin Bran cereal

1 cup (250 mL) skim milk for cereal

1/2 cup (125 mL) calcium-fortified orange juice

tea with 1 tbsp/15 mL milk

- It's a great idea, whenever starting a new eating plan, to use a measuring cup to make sure your serving sizes are correct. For example, measure out 3/4 cup (175 mL) of Raisin Bran so you

Day 2 | Monday

know just what that looks like in your bowl. Keeping your serving sizes in check really does make a difference!

Morning Snack

1 Pumpkin Chocolate Chip Muffin (page 255)
tea with 1 tbsp/15 mL milk

- Don't inhale your food! Eating a snack or meal quickly at your desk or in your car can set you up for a binge. Take time to eat your food and pay attention to every bite.

Lunch

turkey sandwich
2 slices whole-wheat bread
2 oz (60 g) lean turkey
1 tbsp (15 mL) light mayonnaise
6 baby carrots
1 glass (1 cup/250 mL) skim milk
tea with 1 tbsp/15 mL milk

- Most processed luncheon meats are loaded with salt. Use either fresh meat (for example, cold leftover chicken or turkey from a previous dinner) or buy brands of processed meat that are lower in sodium. Schneider's Lifestyle line has over 30% less salt than regular luncheon meats.

Afternoon Snack

16 peanuts
1/4 medium-size cantaloupe

Dinner

1 serving Salmon Chowder (page 223)
1 slice whole-wheat toast
1 tsp (5 mL) nonhydrogenated margarine
water

Dinner or Evening Snack

1 cup (250 mL) chocolate soy milk

- Tasty option: Warm the soy milk in the microwave and top it off with a few mini-marshmallows.

- Don't forget to eliminate the competition. If your kitchen cupboards are filled with cookies and bags of potato chips, chances are you'll be tempted to stray from the Plan.

Day 3 | Tuesday

Breakfast

1 packet instant oatmeal cereal
2 tbsp (25 mL) raisins
1 tbsp (15 mL) ground flaxseed
3/4 cup (175 mL) skim milk for oatmeal (don't use water!)
1/2 cup (125 mL) calcium-fortified orange juice
tea with 1 tbsp/15 mL milk

- Never skip breakfast! It helps kick-start your metabolism (calorie-burning potential) for the day and helps keep your appetite in check.

Morning Snack

3 tbsp (45 mL) roasted soy nuts
tea with 1 tbsp/15 mL milk

Lunch

1 serving Mairlyn's World Famous Beans and Rice (leftover from dinner on Sunday)
1 whole-wheat roll
1 tsp (5 mL) nonhydrogenated margarine
1 glass (1 cup/250 mL) skim milk
tea with 1 tbsp/15 mL milk

12 almonds

6 baby carrots

- Think positive when following a weight-loss plan. Don't focus on what you can't eat. Consider all the wonderful foods you can eat! Healthy eating shouldn't be something you have to do, it should be something you want to do.

1 serving Chicken Burger on Whole-Wheat Bun (page 208)

lettuce and tomato slices on burger (ketchup and mustard are also allowed)

2 cups (500 mL) dark leafy green salad with 2 tbsp (25 mL) Unbelievably Delicious Raspberry Salad Dressing (page 146)

water

1 glass (1 cup/250 mL) skim milk

1/2 M&M's Mini Chocolate Candies tube (30-g tube)

- That's about 50 mini M&M's (if you're counting). If you have the regular size M&M's Chocolate Candies limit yourself to about 20.

- If ever you fall off the plan and indulge in something you know you shouldn't, don't beat yourself up! Simply start anew with the next meal or snack. Research demonstrates that how you handle dietary slips is a very important part of weight-loss success.

Day 4 | Wednesday

1 cup (250 mL) Cheerios cereal

3 tbsp (45 mL) All-Bran Buds cereal

1 cup (250 mL) skim milk for cereal

1/2 cup (125 mL) calcium-fortified orange juice

tea with 1 tbsp/15 mL milk

1 Pumpkin Chocolate Chip Muffin (page 255)

tea with 1 tbsp/15 mL milk

- Don't believe that when you lose weight you will become a wonderful person. You already are a wonderful person!

hummus with pita bread

1 small (4-inch/10-cm) whole-wheat pita bread

1/4 cup (50 mL) Hummus with Roasted Red Peppers (page 229)

1 serving Grape Tomato Salad (page 152)

1 glass (1 cup/250 mL) skim milk

tea with 1 tbsp/15 mL milk

- If you don't have time to make hummus from scratch, buy ready-made hummus. Look for lower fat brands.

- The Grape Tomato Salad can be made the night before.

1 small red pepper, cut into strips

1 tbsp (15 mL) light creamy salad dressing (for dipping)

- Look for salad dressings that are lower in sodium.

Day 4 | Wednesday

1 serving Stir-Fried Broccoli with Cashews (page 174)

1 cup (250 mL) brown rice

1 glass (1 cup/250 mL) skim milk

- This is the perfect example of nuts being used as a replacement to meat in a main course meal.

- It's okay to use bottled marinades or stir-fry sauces when you're in a hurry and want to throw together a quick stir-fry with lots of veggies and some lean meat or poultry. Look for sauces that are low in fat and contain no more than 300 mg sodium per 2 tbsp (25 mL) serving. President's Choice Memories of Mum's Kitchen Soya Ginger is one of my favorites. Safeway Select Cook 'N Grill Plum Sauce is also very good.

Dessert or Evening Snack

1 serving Big Blue Berry Purple Smoothie (page 247)

- Did you remember to exercise today? When you combine a lower calorie diet with regular physical activity, you preserve or increase your lean body mass (muscle) while you lose body fat.

Day 5 | Thursday

Breakfast

2/3 cup (150 mL) Shreddies cereal

1/4 cup (50 mL) All-Bran Buds cereal

1 cup (250 mL) skim milk for cereal

1/2 cup (125 mL) calcium-fortified orange juice

tea with 1 tbsp/15 mL milk

Morning Snack

1 Pumpkin Chocolate Chip Muffin (page 255)

tea with 1 tbsp/15 mL milk

Lunch

tuna salad sandwich

2 slices whole-wheat bread

2 oz (60 g) drained, canned white tuna

1 tbsp (15 mL) light mayonnaise

1/4 cup (50 mL) diced red pepper

tea with 1 tbsp/15 mL milk

- When it comes to tuna, salmon, chicken or turkey salad sandwiches, make your own or get your sandwich made to order with small quantities of light mayo (about 1 tbsp/15 mL). Most food court or restaurant versions of these sandwiches contain regular mayonnaise and usually lots of it.

Afternoon Snack

1 glass (1 cup/250 mL) skim milk

1 kiwi

Dinner

1 serving Salsa Baked Chicken (page 209)

1/2 cup (125 mL) brown rice

1 tsp (5 mL) non-hydrogenated margarine

2 cups (500 mL) dark leafy green salad with 2 tbsp (25 mL) House Dressing (page 145)

water

Dessert or Evening Snack

1 serving Super Chocolate Banana Soy Shake (page 245)

- Don't forget—successful weight management requires a lifelong commitment to healthy eating and regular activity. A good plan is one you can stick with and enjoy along the way!

Day 6 | Friday

3/4 cup (175 mL) Post Fruit & Fibre cereal
1 tbsp (15 mL) ground flaxseed
1 cup (250 mL) skim milk for cereal
1/2 cup (125 mL) calcium-fortified orange juice
tea with 1 tbsp/15 mL milk

- Good news! Research suggests that the longer you maintain a new, lower body weight, the easier it becomes to stay at your new weight.

3 tbsp (45 mL) roasted soy nuts
tea with 1 tbsp/15 mL milk

spinach salad with almonds
2 cups (500 mL) fresh spinach
2 tbsp (25 mL) Unbelievably Delicious Raspberry Dressing (page 146)
12 almonds
1 serving whole-wheat toast
1 tsp (5 mL) nonhydrogenated margarine
1 glass (1 cup/250 mL) skim milk

- One more good reason to drink your milk! Preliminary research suggests that diets high in calcium influence your body's ability to burn fat and make it easier to lose weight.

1 Two-Bite Brownie (available at most super-markets)
tea with 1 tbsp/15 mL milk

- The brownie can be substituted for an alternative chocolate treat as listed in the Leaving Room for Chocolate chapter.

1 serving Rotini with Plum Tomatoes and Lentils (page 190)
6 baby carrots
1 glass (1 cup/250 mL) skim milk

- Some fad diets recommend that people avoid combining certain types of food at the same meal. Reality check: if weight loss is what you're after, it's not how you separate your food that matters but what and how much you eat.

It's Friday, rent a movie and enjoy...
1 glass (5 oz/145 mL) red wine
3 cups (750 mL) light microwave popcorn

- Tasty option: Sprinkle popcorn with cinnamon and either a dusting of icing sugar or a sugar substitute like Splenda.

Day 7 | Saturday

1 cup (250 mL) Cheerios cereal
3 tbsp (45 mL) All-Bran Buds cereal
1 cup (250 mL) skim milk for cereal
1/2 cup (125 mL) calcium-fortified orange juice
tea with 1 tbsp/15 mL milk

1/2 ruby red grapefruit
1 slice whole-wheat toast with 1 tsp (5 mL) jam
tea with 1 tbsp/15 mL milk

1 serving Rotini with Plum Tomatoes and Lentils (leftover from Friday night's dinner)

Day 7 | Saturday

1 glass (1 cup/250 mL) skim milk
tea with 1 tbsp/15 mL milk

- High-protein, low-carbohydrate diets may be popular, but they don't produce lasting results. Based on the National Weight Control Registry in the United States, 99% of people who have lost weight and kept it off, have done so by eating a low-fat, high-carbohydrate diet.

Afternoon Snack

1 Super Soy Strawberry Smoothie (page 247)
1 tbsp (15 mL) ground flaxseed

Dinner

1 serving Company's Comin' Salmon (page 215)
1 serving Brussels Sprouts with Maple Syrup (page 176)
1 serving Wild and Brown Rice (page 179)
1 glass (5 oz/145 mL) red wine

- This is a great dinner to serve to company!

- To earn your glass of wine, go for a walk after dinner.

Dessert or Evening Snack

1 serving Chocolate Fondue (page 269)

- Enjoy with 1/2 cup (125 mL) fresh fruit like strawberries or bananas.

- And who said you can't leave room for chocolate?

Out-of-this-World Delicious Recipes

I have always believed that you are what you eat. I was raised by two parents who believed in eating lots of fruits and vegetables, beans and fish. I thought everybody ate salmon sandwiches for lunch! Mom and Dad grew their own vegetables in the backyard, and some nights we ate all-vegetable meals. I can still see my plate with tomatoes, corn on the cob, beet tops, carrots, green beans, and new potatoes. It was beautiful to look at and delicious to eat. So began my love affair with food!

Some foods can lower your cholesterol, reduce your chances of developing heart disease, and help prevent certain cancers. All this by what you stick in your mouth.

I've always believed that we take better care of our cars and our pets than we do ourselves, and it's time to look to our future and ask ourselves: do we want to be healthy? Do we want to feel as good as we can, have as much energy as we can, and be fit and active till the day we die? I'm answering, yes. A big huge YES!

You've read Liz's section and now you're ready to put the plan into action. Here are my out-of-this-world delicious recipes to help you make that happen.

Mairlyn Smith

Salads

Salad Dressings

Okay, you have committed to eating 5-10 fruits and veggies a day, and having a salad is a great way to add those raw nutrient-packed greens to your diet. You go out and spend money on tons of different types of salad ingredients only to let them turn to slime in the veggie drawer. What's a person to do? Well help is on the way! Go buy a "bag of greens." There are numerous bags of salads out in the market. Look for the baby greens, which are an assortment of tender spring greens, or for the baby spinach greens. Both are terrific to eat and have a good fridge life. Grab a handful of greens, pour on one of these terrific dressings, and you've got one great tasting, easy-to-make salad.

SO WHAT THE HECK DOES UHEP MEAN?
It is the abbreviation for The Ultimate Healthy Eating Plan. Check how many servings of Fat, Soy, Vegetables and Fruit, Fish, etc. you are getting per each serving from the recipe. That way you will be able to count out your daily intake as you eat your way through the book.

House Dressing

My old standby updated to the "Ultimate Healthy" in house dressings. Goes well on all types of greens.

1/4 cup / 60 mL **balsamic vinegar**
1 tbsp + 1 tsp / 20 mL **extra virgin olive oil**
1 tbsp / 15 mL **water**
2 tsp / 10 mL **grainy Dijon mustard** (see page 200)
2 tsp / 10 mL **honey**
1 **clove garlic—crushed**

1   Whisk together all the ingredients. Can be stored up to 1 week in advance.

Makes 1/2 cup/120 mL. Serves 4.

ONE SERVING 2 tbsp/30 mL	58 Calories
	0.2 g protein
	4.9 g fat
	0.1 g fiber
	51 mg sodium
	4 g carbohydrate
UHEP	1 Fat

Unbelievably Delicious Raspberry Salad Dressing

My parents are amazing gardeners. Growing up we had a vegetable garden, a flower garden, a rose garden, and raspberry canes! One of my fondest memories is picking raspberries first thing in the morning in my p.j.'s and plopping them right into my bowl of cereal. They don't get much fresher than that.

Try this wonderful salad dressing, my personal favorite, for a fresh raspberry flavor that tastes like it's right off the cane!

5 tbsp / 75 mL **raspberry cocktail concentrate—thawed**
1 tbsp + 1 tsp / 20 mL **canola oil**
1 **shallot—minced**
1/4 tsp / 1 mL **freshly cracked pepper**
1/4 tsp / 1 mL **paprika**
1/4 tsp / 1 mL **Dijon mustard**

1   Whisk together all the ingredients. Can be stored up to 1 week in advance. Tastes great on a plain green salad with some fresh raspberries thrown in for good measure.

Makes 1/2 cup/120mL. Serves 4.

WHERE DO I FIND RASPBERRY COCKTAIL CONCENTRATE?
It's in the frozen juice aisle at your local grocery store.

WHAT DO I DO WITH THE LEFTOVER RASPBERRY COCKTAIL?
Spoon out the amount that you need in the frozen state and put the rest back in the freezer for the next time you get a raspberry salad dressing attack. Warning—be sure to cover it tightly—spilled frozen raspberry concentrate is really difficult to clean up—words from the voice of experience!

ONE SERVING 2 tbsp/30 mL	55 Calories
	0.2 g protein
	4.6 g fat
	0.1 g fiber
	0.5 mg sodium
	3 g carbohydrate
UHEP	1 Fat

ONE SERVING	58 Calories
Tarragon Vinaigrette	0.1 g protein
	4.7 g fat
	0.2 g fiber
1 tbsp/15 mL	0.3 mg sodium
	5 g carbohydrate
UHEP	1 Fat

Tarragon Vinaigrette

A zesty salad dressing with strong clean flavors.

1 tbsp + 1 tsp / 20 mL **extra virgin olive oil**
1 tbsp + 1 tsp / 20 mL **red wine vinegar**
1 tbsp / 15 mL **honey**
1/2 tsp / 2 mL **dried basil**
1/4 tsp / 1 mL **paprika**
1/4 tsp / 1 mL **dried tarragon**
1/4 tsp / 1 mL **freshly cracked pepper**

1   Whisk together all the ingredients. Can be stored up to 1 week in advance.

Makes 1/4 cup/60 mL. Serves 4.

WHAT THE HECK IS MANGO CHUTNEY AND WHERE DO I FIND IT?

Chutney is an Indian condiment that is like a spicy jam! It goes great with curry, poultry and meat dishes. The mango flavor is wonderful in this salad dressing, but if you can't find it in the condiment aisle try another flavor of chutney.

ONE SERVING	78 Calories
Mango Chutney Dressing	0.1 g protein
	4.7 g fat
	0.2 g fiber
	147 mg sodium
3 tbsp/45 mL	10 g carbohydrate
UHEP	1 Fat

Mango Chutney Dressing

If you are looking for a really different salad dressing, your search is over. This is unique and totally zippy. You are probably thinking that you are never going to try it—but you'd be missing out on a really wonderful taste experience. Give it a go!

3 tbsp / 45 mL **mango chutney**
2 tbsp / 30 mL **lemon juice**
2 tbsp / 30 mL **apple cider vinegar**
1 tbsp + 1 tsp / 20 mL **extra virgin olive oil**
1 tsp / 5 mL **honey**
1/2 tsp / 2 mL **curry powder**
pinch **cayenne**

1   Purée all the ingredients. Can be stored up to 1 week in advance.

Makes 3/4 cup/180 mL. Serves 4.

Strawberry and Spinach Salad

If I were stranded on a deserted island, like Tom Hanks in *Castaway*, I would be craving my cell phone, a chocolate bar, a Boy Scout with matches, and this salad.

8 cups / 2 L **baby spinach**
24 / about 3 cups **strawberries**
1/2 cup / 125 mL **chopped almonds—optional**

Dressing
2 tbsp + 2 tsp / 35 mL **extra virgin olive oil**
2 tbsp + 2 tsp / 35 mL **balsamic vinegar**
2 tbsp / 25 mL **dark brown sugar**
2 tbsp / 25 mL **raspberry concentrate** (see page 146)
1/2 tsp / 2 mL **paprika**
1/2 tsp / 2 mL **Worcestershire sauce**

1   Wash and dry the spinach. Store wrapped in a paper towel in a plastic bag in the fridge till ready to use.

2   Wash the strawberries and lay out on a cloth or paper towels to let dry.

3   In a small bowl, whisk together the olive oil, balsamic vinegar, sugar, raspberry concentrate, paprika and Worcestershire sauce. Set aside till serving time.

4   Hull and slice the strawberries. Set aside until serving time.

5   Serving time! You have 2 serving choices.

   1   Divide the spinach equally among the 4 plates, sprinkle equally with the sliced strawberries, then sprinkle with 1/4 of the salad dressing and top with 2 tbsp/25 mL of the chopped almonds (if using).

   2   Toss everything together in a bowl and then divide equally among the 4 plates.

   Serves 4.

ONE SERVING without almonds	145 Calories
	2.2 g protein
	9.8 g fat
	3.4 g fiber
	57 mg sodium
	15 g carbohydrate
UHEP	2 Fat
	3 Vegetables & Fruit

ONE SERVING with almonds	214 Calories
	4.7 g protein
	15.8 g fat
	4.8 g fiber
	57 mg sodium
	17 g carbohydrate
UHEP	2 Fat
	3 Vegetables & Fruit
	1/2 Nuts

Romaine with Feta and Blueberries

DINNER PARTY

You can prep this salad in advance, making it a great choice for a dinner party.

I started making this salad the summer I bought a ton of wild blueberries on my way home from a day in the country. I made blueberry muffins and pancakes till they were coming out of our ears! I was going to freeze the rest when I got the culinary notion to toss them with feta. Sounds weird, tastes great.

1 **large head of romaine**
2 cups / 500 mL **wild blueberries**

Dressing
1/3 cup / 75 mL **light feta cheese**
1/4 cup / 50 mL **apple cider vinegar**
1 tbsp + 1 tsp / 20 mL **extra virgin olive oil**
1 **shallot**
1 tbsp / 15 mL **honey**

1   Wash romaine, spin dry and wrap in paper towels. It can be placed into a plastic bag and stored in the fridge for up to 2 days.

2   Wash blueberries. Drain well and dry. They can be stored in the fridge for up to 2 days.

3   Using a hand blender, or mini food processor, purée feta, cider vinegar, olive oil, shallot and honey. It can be stored in fridge for up to 2 days.

4   Serving time—tear or chop romaine into bite-sized pieces, toss in a large bowl with the salad dressing.

5   Add blueberries, toss and serve.

Serves 4

ONE SERVING	145 Calories
with 2 tbsp/25 mL of dressing	3.7 g protein
	7.2 g fat
	2.7 g fiber
	19 mg sodium
	19 g carbohydrate
UHEP	1 Fat
	2 Vegetables & Fruit
	1/4 Milk

Spinach Salad

I took the idea of apples and walnuts from the traditional Waldorf Salad and blended it with the original idea of adding spinach, red pepper, and salad dressing. Removing half the fat from the salad dressing using yogurt, was my assistant, Dawn's, idea. Just goes to show you two heads are better than one!

8 cups / 2 L **baby spinach**
2 **red peppers—julienned**
1 **large Granny Smith apple—chopped into 16 slices**
1/2 cup / 125 mL **walnuts—chopped**

Dressing
2 tbsp / 25 mL **low-fat mayonnaise**
2 tbsp / 25 mL **low-fat plain yogurt**
2 tbsp / 25 mL **cider vinegar**
1 tbsp / 15 mL **maple syrup**

1 Wash and spin dry the spinach, unless you took my advice and bought a package of prewashed baby spinach greens.

2 Whisk together the dressing ingredients. Toss the spinach, red pepper and apple with the dressing.

3 Divide the salad equally among 4 plates. Sprinkle each plate with 2 tbsp/25 mL of the walnuts. Serve to rave reviews.

Serves 4

ONE SERVING	213 Calories
	6.9 g protein
	13.1 g fat
	5.6 g fiber
	55 mg sodium
	20 g carbohydrate
UHEP	1/2 Fat
	2 1/2 Vegetables & Fruit
	1/2 Nuts

2/10
no good

Carrot Salad

I have always been a big fan of the lowly carrot. My dad grew them in his famous vegetable garden, I dabbled in its juice in the '70s and I pack the baby ones in my son's lunch.

If I had to choose just one vegetable to live on, carrots would be in my top five list. They are easy to find in the grocery store, never go out of season, can be steamed, stir-fried, eaten raw, baked in a cake or mixed in a salad! What a versatile little orange veggie!

4 **large carrots**
2 tsp / 10 mL **finely grated fresh ginger**
1 tbsp + 1 tsp / 20 mL **low-fat mayonnaise**
1 tbsp + 1 tsp / 20 mL **low-fat plain yogurt**
2 tbsp / 25 mL **mango chutney**
1/4 cup / 50 mL **raisins**
1/4 cup / 50 mL **chopped walnuts**

1   Lightly scrape off the peel of the carrots. Grate carrots into a bowl.

2   Mix in the grated ginger, low-fat mayonnaise, low-fat yogurt, mango chutney, raisins and walnuts.

3   Serve right away or store in the fridge for up to 2 days.

Serves 6

ONE SERVING	101 Calories
	1.9 g protein
	4.4 g fat
	2.5 g fiber
	86 mg sodium
	15 g carbohydrate
UHEP	1 1/2 Vegetables & Fruit

Grape Tomato Salad

In the middle of winter somehow tomatoes just don't taste like tomatoes. Enter the newest tomato in the "love apple" category—Grape Tomatoes! These tiny tomatoes are smaller and sweeter than cherry tomatoes and are available all year long. I love them in this salad, they keep their shape well and the flavors are truly summertime any time of year.

NO GRAPE TOMATOES?
Feel free to use cherry tomatoes. Cut them into quarters.

NOTE TO THE OLIVE-CHALLENGED
Yes, you can omit them.

2 cups / 500 mL **grape tomatoes, cut in halves**
1 tbsp + 1 tsp / 20 mL **extra virgin olive oil**
1 **clove garlic—minced**
10 **fresh basil leaves—chopped**
6 **green olives—diced**
pinch **hot pepper flakes**

1   Mix together all the ingredients in a medium bowl. Let sit for at least 1 hour. Serve over lettuce or eat alone as a vegetable side dish. Can be stored in the fridge for at least 2 days.

Serves 4

ONE SERVING with olives	68 Calories
	0.9 g protein
	5.7 g fat
	1.3 g fiber
	65 mg sodium
	5 g carbohydrate
UHEP	1 Fat
	1 Vegetables & Fruit
ONE SERVING without olives	60 Calories
	0.9 g protein
	5.0 g fat
	1.1 g fiber
	8 mg sodium
	4 g carbohydrate
UHEP	1 Fat
	1 Vegetables & Fruit

Soups

Broccoli Soup

If broccoli is not a standard green vegetable that crosses your doorstep, then this is the recipe for you. It's a very "friendly" recipe, not too green, not too broccoli tasting, and not too hard to prepare. This is what we call a "hat trick" at my house. Am I a hockey mom or what?

3 cups / 750 mL **vegetable stock or lower-sodium chicken stock**
1 cup / 250 mL **water**
1 **onion—diced**
2 **cloves garlic—minced**
4 cups / 1 L **chopped broccoli**
3/4 cup / 175 mL **fat-free evaporated milk**
1/4 tsp / 1 mL **white pepper**

1   In a medium-sized pot, stir together the vegetable stock, water, onion, garlic and broccoli. Bring to a boil. Reduce to simmer, cover and continue simmering until the broccoli and onions are soft, about 20 to 25 minutes.

2   Purée the soup, using a hand-held blender, free-standing blender, or a food processor. Continue on or refrigerate for up to 3 days.

3   Reheat, if necessary, and add the milk. Season with the pepper. Serve immediately.

Serves 6

WHY YOU NEED A HAND-HELD BLENDER

Instead of pouring hot soup into a blender and then making a huge mess because you filled it too high and it exploded all over the wall, all you do is put the hand held blender into the pot and turn it on. It's easy, handy and wonderful. I have one. You need one. Ask for it as a gift. They range anywhere from $45–$75 It is one of the few things that I wouldn't give up, bearing in mind that I did give up two husbands.

ONE SERVING	66 Calories
	4.8 g protein
vegetable stock	0.4 g fat
	2.4 g fiber
	410 mg sodium
	12 g carbohydrate
lower-sodium chicken stock	357 mg sodium
regular chicken stock	543 mg sodium
UHEP	1 1/4 Vegetables & Fruit

Chicken Stock

CHICKEN STOCK: TWO WAYS TO MAKE IT. YOUR PICK!

1. Go to the grocery store and buy a can or tetra pak carton of regular chicken stock or lower-sodium chicken stock.

OR

2. Simmer a chicken in a large pot of water to which you have added 2 carrots, 1 onion, 1 stalk celery and 3 cloves of garlic. Simmer for at least 4 hours. Cool. Remove the chicken. Remove the skin and meat from the chicken and save for a soup recipe or something else. Pour the cooled broth into a container. Put in the fridge overnight. The next day, skim off all the fat from the top of the broth. Use in any recipe calling for chicken stock.

May I Have Your Attention, Please. Chicken Stock—Homemade vs Regular Canned and Lower-sodium Canned—The Great Salt Debate

- Homemade chicken stock is low in sodium as long as you don't add any salt to it.

- Regular canned chicken stock is high in sodium, on average 910 mg per cup.

- Lower-sodium canned chicken stock contains less sodium than regular, on average 600 mg per cup.

About 3% of the population makes their own chicken stock. I'm not one of them. I use lower-sodium chicken stock or vegetable stock which has on average 710 mg of sodium per cup. It is recommended that you limit your sodium intake to 2400 mg/day or less.

The Ultimate Healthy Eating Plan has less than 2400 mg/day. Thank you for your attention.

7/10
— chop tomatoes up small

Marvelous Minestrone

This is a quick and easy all-in-one meal. It's packed with outstanding veggies, like tomatoes, carrots, onions and kale, whole-grain pasta, healthy extra virgin olive oil and cholesterol-lowering beans! I made this on CBC's *Newsworld* one morning and the crew gobbled it up! A true testimonial—eating beans at 8 a.m.

KID-FRIENDLY TIP
Skip the pepper and the red pepper flakes. Add them to the adults' soup when serving. Sprinkle kids' with a bit more cheese.

1 tbsp + 1 tsp / 20 mL **extra virgin olive oil**
1 **large onion—diced**
2 **large carrots—chopped**
4 **cloves garlic—minced**
1 28-oz / /96-mL can **plum tomatoes**
1 19-oz / 540-mL can **kidney beans—rinsed and drained**
2 cups / 500 mL **vegetable stock or lower-sodium chicken stock**
1 1/2 cups / 375 mL **water**
4 cups / 1 L **kale** (see page 181)
1/2 cup / 125 mL **whole-wheat rotini**
1/4 tsp / 1 mL **pepper**
1/2 tsp / 2 mL **red pepper flakes**
2 tbsp / 25 mL **chopped fresh basil**

1 Heat the oil in a large pot.

2 Add the onion and sauté till almost cooked, about 5 minutes, stirring often.

3 Add the carrots and the garlic. Sauté for 3 minutes, stirring often.

4 Add the plum tomatoes, kidney beans and stock. Chop up the tomatoes slightly. Remove kale from stalks. Discard stalks. Chop kale leaves.

5 Bring to the boil. Add the kale, whole-wheat rotini, pepper and red pepper flakes. Bring back to the boil. Reduce heat to simmer. Cover and cook for 10 to 12 minutes or until the pasta is cooked.

6 Add the basil and serve. If desired, sprinkle with Parmesan cheese.

Serves 6

ONE SERVING	224 Calories
vegetable stock	9.8 g protein
	4.4 g fat
	12.1 g fiber
	722 mg sodium
	38 g carbohydrate
lower-sodium chicken stock	687 mg sodium
regular chicken stock	811 mg sodium
UHEP	3/4 Beans
	3/4 Fat
	2 1/2 Vegetables & Fruit
	1/4 Grains

Quick and Hearty Chicken Noodle Soup

Kid-Approved

Nothing beats a hot bowl of chicken soup when you have a cold. The vapors help unplug your sinuses and the nostalgia of eating homemade soup will make you feel better, at least emotionally. It's like a big warm hug all in a bowl!

4 cups / 1 L **chicken stock or lower-sodium chicken stock**
1 **onion—minced**
3 **cloves garlic—minced**
2 **large carrots—diced**
2 cups / 500 mL **kale** (see page 181)
1 cup / 250 mL **whole-wheat rotini**
14 oz / 400 g **skinless boneless chicken breast**

1   Pour the chicken stock into a medium saucepan.

2   Turn the heat to high. Add the onion and garlic to the stock.

3   Add the carrots.

4   Wash the kale and then remove the leaves from the stalk. The stalk tends to make the kale taste bitter, so don't use it!

5   Chop the kale up to make 2 cups/500 mL. This will probably take about 4 to 6 leaves of kale.

6   Chop up the chicken into 1-in/2.5-cm pieces.

7   When the stock has come to the boil, add the kale, rotini and chicken. Return to the boil, then lower the heat to simmer, cover and cook for 10 minutes or until chicken is cooked.

8   Serve.

Serves 4

ONE SERVING	293 Calories
	37.2 g protein
	4.4 g fat
	3.4 g fiber
	1068 mg sodium
	25 g carbohydrate
lower-sodium chicken stock	696 mg sodium
UHEP	1 3/4 Vegetables & Fruit
	1 Grains
	1 Meat

Lentil Soup

A great soup that is easy and delicious using the mighty "little" lentil.

2 cups / 500 mL **vegetable stock or lower-sodium chicken stock**
1 cup / 250 mL **water**
1 **onion—diced**
1 **sweet potato—peeled and diced**
2 **carrots—diced**
2 **stalks celery—diced**
1 19-oz / 540-mL can **lentils—drained and rinsed**
1/2 tsp / 2 mL **cumin**

1   Put all the ingredients into a medium pot. Bring to the boil. Cover and simmer for 20 minutes or until the onions are soft.

2   Purée. Serve. Easy.

Serves 6

ONE SERVING	128 Calories
	7.3 g protein
vegetable stock	0.5 g fat
	4.4 g fiber
	412 mg sodium
	25 g carbohydrate
lower-sodium chicken stock	377 mg sodium
regular chicken stock	501 mg sodium
UHEP	3/4 Beans
	1 Vegetables & Fruit

Black Bean Soup

KID-FRIENDLY TIP

Most kids don't like cold yogurt floating in their hot soup! So omit the yogurt and the cilantro. For that matter, a lot of adults don't like cilantro or cold yogurt in hot soup either! Ask first. It still tastes great without it.

This is a wonderful soup for a cold winter's night. The fresh lime really adds that extra special flavor, so don't even think about leaving it out! I like to serve it with whole-wheat toast and a green salad with my Unbelievably Delicious Raspberry Salad Dressing on page 146.

2 cups / 500 mL **vegetable broth or lower-sodium chicken stock**
1 cup / 250 mL **water**
4 **cloves garlic—crushed**
1 **medium onion—diced**
1 **large red pepper—diced**
1 19-oz / 540-mL can **black beans—drained and rinsed**
2 tsp / 10 mL **cumin**
1 tsp / 5 mL **coriander**
1/2 **a lime—juice of**
1/2 cup / 125 mL **low-fat plain yogurt—optional**
1/4 cup / 50 mL **fresh cilantro—minced—optional**

1 In a medium pot mix together the broth or stock, water, garlic, onion and red pepper. Bring to the boil.

2 Add the black beans, cumin and coriander. Stir.

3 Cover and simmer for 20 to 25 minutes or until the onion and red pepper are soft.

4 Purée the soup.

5 Add the juice from the 1/2 lime. Mix well.

6 If using, serve each bowl with 2 tbsp/25 mL of low-fat yogurt and 1 tbsp/15 mL of the minced fresh cilantro.

Serves 4

ONE SERVING	173 Calories
vegetable stock	10.0 g protein
	1.0 g fat
	10.1 g fiber
	473 mg sodium
	33 g carbohydrate
lower-sodium chicken stock	420 mg sodium
regular chicken stock	606 mg sodium

ONE SERVING	192 Calories
vegetable stock with yogurt and cilantro	11.5 g protein
	1.4 g fat
	10.1 g fiber
	496 mg sodium
	35 g carbohydrate
lower-sodium chicken stock	443 mg sodium
regular chicken stock	629 mg sodium

UHEP	1 Beans
	1/2 Vegetables & Fruit

6/10

Skinny Squash Soup

Kid-Approved

The most challenging part about cooking a winter squash is cutting through its hard, thick skin. You have several choices here—throw it at the wall, use a cleaver and hope that you are a good aim, or bake it whole. This method, although not as exciting, is by far the least perilous.

1 **large butternut squash—approx. 4 lb / 2 kg**
1 tbsp + 1 tsp / 20 mL **extra virgin olive oil**
2 **medium onions—diced**
3 1/2 cups / 875 mL **chicken stock or lower-sodium chicken stock**
1 **pear—peeled and diced**
1/2 cup / 125 mL **orange juice**

1 Preheat oven to 350°F/175°C. Wash the squash and pierce with a fork.

2 Place the squash onto a baking pan lined with parchment paper. Roast until cooked, approx. 2 hours.

3 Remove from oven and cool. This can be done the day before you make the soup.

4 When cool enough to handle, cut the squash in half, scrape out the seeds, and scoop out the pulp.

5 In a large pot, heat the oil, sauté the onion. Add the stock and the cooked squash. Bring to the boil. Cover and reduce to simmer. Cook until the onions are soft, approx. 10 to 15 minutes.

6 Add the diced pear. Simmer until cooked, about 5 minutes.

7 Add the orange juice. Heat through.

8 Purée soup using a hand-held blender, a free-standing blender or a food processor. Serve.

Serves 6

SPEEDY TIP
You can always microwave the squash instead of baking it. Follow steps 1 to 4, but don't turn on the oven, use the microwave. It will take about 10 to 20 minutes to cook it, depending on the size of the squash and the age of your microwave. You see, it always comes down to age!

ONE SERVING	125 Calories
	3.7 g protein
	3.6 g fat
	3.7 g fiber
	581 mg sodium
	23 g carbohydrate
lower-sodium chicken stock	364 mg sodium
UHEP	3/4 Fat
	1 1/2 Vegetables & Fruit

Gazpacho

KID-FRIENDLY TIP

Quite frankly, most kids don't like this at all. Offer a taste—if they don't like it, have a plate of chopped red peppers and cucumbers ready. But always offer it first, before you tell them that you have made something else as well.

I never liked cold soup as a kid. It just seemed too weird to have a bowl of something cold that wasn't sweet like, say, ice cream. Savory food in a bowl should be hot. Kid rules! Well, then I moved from "lovely cool summers Vancouver" to "fry an egg on the sidewalk summers Toronto," and suddenly, cold, savory, gazpacho tasted great on a hot humid day.

2 1/2 lb / 1.1 kg **ripe tomatoes, preferably beefsteak—about 8**
1 **large English cucumber**
1 **red pepper**
1 **clove garlic—minced**
2 tsp / 10 mL **extra virgin olive oil**
1/4 cup / 50 mL **red wine vinegar**
1 cup / 250 mL **V8 juice or another type of vegetable juice**
1 cup / 250 mL **chicken stock or lower-sodium chicken stock**
1 tbsp / 15 mL **Worcestershire sauce**
freshly ground pepper
1/4 cup / 50 mL **finely minced chives—for garnish**

1   Chop the tomatoes, cucumber and red pepper into approximately 1/4-in/0.6-cm pieces. Place in a large bowl.

2   Add all the rest of the ingredients except the chives.

3   Refrigerate for at least 8 hours or overnight.

4   Serve garnished with chives.

Serves 8

ONE SERVING	60 Calories
	2.1 g protein
	1.8 g fat
	2.4 g fiber
	167 mg sodium
	11 g carbohydrate
lower-sodium chicken stock	120 mg sodium
UHEP	1/4 Fat
	1 Vegetables & Fruit

Veggies

Quick Vegetable Side Dishes

The next 4 recipes are quick and easy vegetable side dishes that you can whip up in about 5 minutes.

Honey Glazed Carrots
Kid-Approved

This recipe is for Liz! She loves carrots served this way and so do her two daughters. Well, since I tried them out at home they are a favorite of ours as well. I use the peeled baby carrots. All you have to do is take them out of the package and steam them! Simple, and a great way to encourage non-veggies-lovers to eat their orange vegetables.

ONE SERVING	67 Calories 0.6 g protein 3.0 g fat 1.8 g fiber 39 mg sodium 10 g carbohydrate
UHEP	3/4 Fat 1 Vegetables & Fruit

2 cups / 500 mL **baby carrots**
1 tbsp / 15 mL **nonhydrogenated margarine**
1 tbsp / 15 mL **honey**

1   Steam carrots till tender-crisp, about 3 to 5 minutes.

2   Drain. Add the nonhydrogenated margarine and honey. Heat until bubbly. Serve.

Serves 4

Honey Dijon Glazed Carrots
An adult version of the theme.

6/16

ONE SERVING	68 Calories 0.6 g protein 3.0 g fat 1.8 g fiber 39 mg sodium 10 g carbohydrate
UHEP	3/4 Fat 1 Vegetables & Fruit

2 cups / 500 mL **baby carrots**
1 tbsp / 15 mL **nonhydrogenated margarine**
1 tbsp / 15 mL **honey**
1 tsp / 5 mL **Dijon mustard**

1   Steam carrots till tender-crisp, about 3 to 5 minutes.

2   Drain. Add the nonhydrogenated margarine, honey and Dijon. Heat until bubbly. Serve.

Serves 4

Quick Vegetable Side Dishes (cont.)

Tomatoes with Fresh Basil

My parents are excellent gardeners. They were composting back in the '50s before the term environmentally-friendly had even been coined. Talk about your trendsetters. That composter was the size of an Austin mini—I ought to know, since I once took a dare and jumped off the garage roof right into it. Unscathed I might add.

They fertilized with the compost and grew fantastic vegetables, making them famous in the neighborhood. Their forte was tomatoes, huge beefsteak tomatoes. I can still taste them. This recipe reminds me of my parents and their vegetable garden. Cheers to Mom and Dad.

3 **large ripe beefsteak tomatoes—at room temperature**
1 **small clove garlic—crushed**
2 tsp / 10 mL **extra virgin olive oil**
1 tbsp / 15 mL **balsamic vinegar**
1/2 cup / 125 mL **loosely packed fresh basil—sliced thinly**

1 Slice the tomatoes into 1/2-in/1.2-cm slices. Lay them on a plate.

2 Mix together the garlic, olive oil and balsamic vinegar. Drizzle over the tomatoes. Sprinkle with the basil.

3 Let stand for 30 minutes. Serve.

Serves 4

ONE SERVING	33 Calories
	0.6 g protein
	2.5 g fat
	0.7 g fiber
	4 mg sodium
	3 g carbohydrate
UHEP	1/2 Fat
	1 Vegetables & Fruit

ONE SERVING	94 Calories
	1.5 g protein
	0.2 g fat
	1.4 g fiber
	10 mg sodium
	22 g carbohydrate
UHEP	1 Vegetables & Fruit

Quickie Sweet Potatoes

Sweet potatoes are often called yams in the produce section. This is totally incorrect. I tried explaining the difference between sweet potatoes and yams to the produce manager at my local grocery store—he now thinks I am a total whacko!

A sweet potato bears about as much resemblance to a yam as I do to a Rockette! All sweet potatoes have yellow-orange to red-orange flesh. A yam on the other hand has white flesh. Two totally different interiors! Me and a Rockette—two totally different exteriors.

One of these days I am going to take a sweet potato and a yam over to "Mr. I Am the Big Produce Guy" and give him a little botanical lesson!

2 **medium sweet potatoes**
2–3 tbsp / 25–45 mL **frozen concentrated orange juice, thawed**

1   Scrub the sweet potatoes and prick them with a fork.

2   Microwave on high for 10 to 12 minutes, depending on their size.

3   Once they are soft, let them rest in a bowl for 5 minutes.

4   This little "sweet potato rest time" makes it easy to skin them, which just happens to be the next step. Skin sweet potatoes.

5   Mash the sweet potatoes together with 2 tbsp/25 mL of the orange juice concentrate.

6   For a more intense orange flavor, add one more table-spoon (15 mL) of concentrate.

Serves 4

Three Squash Quickies

Here are 3 winter squash recipes that are all cooked in the microwave and are ready in 10 to 15 minutes.

Acorn Squash with Maple Syrup

This dark green- or orange-skinned squash is shaped like a really big acorn! An acorn about the size of a cabbage. Imagine how big the squirrels would be if they had to store a couple of these every winter!

For some reason it is sometimes called a pepper squash which has nothing to do with what it looks like. Just when you think you know the answers, someone changes the rules.

1 **acorn or pepper squash**
2 tsp / 10 mL **nonhydrogenated margarine**
2 tsp / 10 mL **maple syrup**
1/4 cup / 50 mL **water**

1   Cut the squash into quarters. Scoop out the seeds.

2   Place the squash into a microwave-safe casserole dish. Dot with the margarine and maple syrup. Add 1/4 cup/ 50 mL water to the bottom of the dish. Cover and microwave on high for 10 to 12 minutes or until soft. Serve.

Serves 4

ONE SERVING	66 Calories
	1.6 g protein
	2.2 g fat
	1.6 g fiber
	17 mg sodium
	12 g carbohydrate
UHEP	1/2 Fat
	1 Vegetables & Fruit

Butternut Squash with Brown Sugar and Cinnamon

This sweet smooth squash is by far most people's favorite. It has a wonderful creamy quality when cooked. It looks a bit like a lopsided dumbbell (no, not that produce guy that I'm always talking about—a weight)!

2 lb / 900 g **butternut squash**
2 tsp / 10 mL **nonhydrogenated margarine**
2 tsp / 10 mL **brown sugar**
1 tsp / 5 mL **cinnamon**

1   Using a large knife cut the squash into quarters. Scoop out the seeds.

2   Place the butternut squash into a microwave-safe casserole dish. Dot with the margarine and the brown sugar. Microwave on high for 10 to 15 minutes or until soft.

3   When cooked through, scoop out the flesh and mash. Sprinkle with cinnamon.

Serves 4

ONE SERVING	73 Calories
	2.2 g protein
	1.7 g fat
	2.5 g fiber
	15 mg sodium
	15 g carbohydrate
UHEP	1/2 Fat
	1 Vegetables & Fruit

Sweet Spaghetti Squash

This squash looks like a yellow football. When cooked the flesh turns into spaghetti-like strands! Some people pour tomato sauce over it, but I prefer the usual—margarine and a sweetener.

1 **spaghetti squash**
2 tsp / 10 mL **nonhydrogenated margarine**
1 tsp / 5 mL **honey**

1 Using a large knife cut the spaghetti squash in half. Store the other half in the fridge for up to 5 days.

2 Place the spaghetti squash into a microwave-safe casserole dish. Add 2/3 cup/150 mL water and cover. Microwave on high for 10 to 15 minutes.

3 Using a fork, shred the flesh.

4 Toss with the margarine and honey. Serve.

Serves 4. Makes 2 cups/500 mL cooked.

ONE SERVING	43 Calories
	0.8 g protein
	2.1 g fat
	0.8 g fiber
	15 mg sodium
	6 g carbohydrate
UHEP	1/2 Fat
	1 Vegetables & Fruit

Grilled Veggie Salad

GRILLING TIP

Don't be tempted to cut the peppers into small pieces before you grill them—they fall through the grill! Been there, done that! Or you can buy one of those really great grill pans and cut the veggies up, then grill.

I make this grilled salad every summer up at my friend's cottage. It is so simple, especially if you get someone else to stand over the hot coals while you lounge by the lake sipping a cool cocktail. Wine spritzers are especially delightful.

1 **red pepper—cut into quarters**
1 **orange pepper—cut into quarters**
1 **green pepper—cut into quarters**
1 **Vidalia onion or sweet onion—cut into 6 slices**
8 **mushrooms**
1 tsp / 5 mL **extra virgin olive oil**

Dressing
2 tbsp / 25 mL **balsamic vinegar**
2 tsp / 10 mL **extra virgin olive oil**
1 tsp / 5 mL **grainy Dijon mustard**
1 tsp / 5 mL **honey**
1 **small clove garlic—crushed**

1   In a large bowl, toss the veggies with the 1 tsp of olive oil.

2   Grill until slightly blackened.

3   Cut each cooked pepper into 4 pieces.

4   Whisk dressing ingredients together. Toss in the veggies. Serve at room temperature.

Serves 4

ONE SERVING	86 Calories
	2.5 g protein
	3.9 g fat
	2.6 g fiber
	30 mg sodium
	13 g carbohydrate
UHEP	3/4 Fat
	1 1/2 Vegetables & Fruit

Yellow and Red Peppers
with Vidalia Onions

Vidalia onions are a sweet onion that you can eat like an apple although your breath is nothing like apple afterwards! Vidalias are grown in the state of Georgia, and most Easterners are familiar with them as they first appear in the produce section in May. On the west coast consumers usually see Walla Wallas from the state of Washington right around the same time of year. If you can't get either kind, move, or use a Spanish onion.

1 tbsp + 1 tsp / 20 mL **extra virgin olive oil**
1 **large Vidalia onion—thinly sliced**
2 **medium sweet yellow peppers—thinly sliced**
2 **medium sweet red peppers—thinly sliced**
1 tbsp / 15 mL **balsamic vinegar**

1   Heat a large frying pan. Add the olive oil.

2   Add the onion and sauté until almost translucent, about 3 to 4 minutes.

3   Add the yellow and red pepper strips and sauté for 2 more minutes or until hot and tender-crisp.

4   Add the balsamic vinegar and sauté for 30 seconds. Serve.

Serves 6

ONE SERVING	68 Calories
	1.4 g protein
	3.4 g fat
	1.9 g fiber
	3 mg sodium
	10 g carbohydrate
UHEP	3/4 Fat
	1 Vegetables & Fruit

Oven Roasted Sweet Potatoes x 2

Kid-Approved

SO WHAT THE HECK IS PARCHMENT PAPER?

It is a nonstick cooking paper that goes into the oven without burning or letting anything stick to it! It really speeds up cleanup and in some cases you don't have anything to clean up. I haven't washed my cookie sheet since I started using it! You can find it with all the other papers in the grocery store. It's usually beside, or really close to, the wax paper, speaking of which, don't use wax paper instead. It smokes and melts! Buy the parchment paper. The one that I use is Chef's Select.

No parchment paper? Jump in your car, drive to your nearest grocery store, and buy a ton! If this isn't an option then make a mental note to buy parchment paper the next time you are grocery shopping. You'll thank me for it.

I started roasting sweet potatoes when Andrew, my son, was two years old. I thought to myself, if potatoes taste great using this method, so would sweet potatoes. I was right. Sometimes it's so hard to be humble! Andrew ate so many sweet potatoes over the course of two weeks he started turning orange! Too much of a good thing! We cut back and dabbled in broccoli.

Here are two different recipes that I use all the time. The method is the same for both, so go nuts, try them both!

Honey Lime Sweet Potatoes—Recipe 1

2 **sweet potatoes—peeled and sliced into 1/4-in/0.6-cm coins**
2 **tsp / 10 mL extra virgin olive oil**
1 **lime—juice of**
2 tbsp / 25 mL **honey**

Sweet Potato Coins—Recipe 2

2 **sweet potatoes—peeled and sliced into 1/4-in/0.6-cm coins**
1 tbsp + 1 tsp / 20 mL **extra virgin olive oil**
1 tsp / 5 mL **onion powder**
1 tsp / 5 mL **garlic powder**
1 tsp / 5 mL **paprika**
1/4 tsp / 1 mL **cumin**

1 Preheat the oven to 425°F/220°C.

2 Line a cookie sheet with parchment paper or foil.

3 Toss the sweet potatoes in the mixture in Recipe #1 or Recipe #2. Spread out in the prepared sheet.

4 Roast for 15 minutes. Flip over. Continue roasting for another 15 minutes. Check to see that they are cooked right through.

5 Serve.

Serves 4

ONE SERVING Honey Lime Sweet Potatoes	134 Calories 1.3 g protein 2.6 g fat 1.4 g fiber 10 mg sodium 27 g carbohydrate
UHEP	1/2 Fat 1 Vegetables & Fruit
ONE SERVING Sweet Potato Coins	128 Calories 1.6 g protein 5.3 g fat 1.7 g fiber 11 mg sodium 20 g carbohydrate
UHEP	1 Fat 1 Vegetables & Fruit

10/10 ! Matt "would eat it every day"

Asparagus with Balsamic Vinegar

I wait for the local asparagus to hit the produce aisle before I start buying it. I love to support my local farmers, and filling up on their produce is one great way to help your community while helping yourself get those all-powerful 5–10 fruits and veggies a day.

1 lb / 450 g **asparagus—about 24 stalks**
1/2 **red pepper—diced**
1 tbsp / 15 mL **balsamic vinegar**
1/2 cup / 125 mL **chicken stock or lower-sodium chicken stock—in 2 portions**
1 tsp / 5 mL **cornstarch**
2 tsp / 10 mL **extra virgin olive oil**

1   Wash the asparagus. Remove the tough stems. Cut the remaining asparagus into 3 equal lengths. Set aside.

2   Mix together the balsamic vinegar, 1/4 cup/50 mL of the chicken stock and the cornstarch. Set aside.

3   Heat a nonstick pan. Add the oil. Add the asparagus and the red pepper. Sauté. Add the remaining chicken stock and continue sautéing until the asparagus is tender-crisp.

4   Stir in the balsamic vinegar mixture and cook until the sauce thickens. Serve.

Serves 4

ONE SERVING	58 Calories
	4.2 g protein
	2.4 g fat
	2.1 g fiber
	126 mg sodium
	8 g carbohydrate
lower-sodium chicken stock	78 mg sodium
UHEP	1/2 Fat
	1 Vegetables & Fruit

Broccoli, Red Pepper and Fresh Ginger

Here is a fast and easy way to serve that powerhouse of veggies—the true green giant of the vegetable world—broccoli.

1 tbsp / 15 mL **extra virgin olive oil**
4 cups / 1 L **broccoli florets**
1 tsp / 5 mL **grated fresh ginger**
1/4 cup / 50 mL **water**
1 **large sweet red pepper—cut into strips**

1 Heat a large frying pan or wok. Add the olive oil.

2 Add the broccoli. Stir-fry for 1 to 2 minutes.

3 Add the ginger and water. Put on the lid and cook for 2 to 3 minutes.

4 Add the red pepper, toss. Cover and cook for 1 to 2 more minutes. Serve immediately.

Serves 4

ONE SERVING	61 Calories
	2.5 g protein
	3.8 g fat
	3.5 g fiber
	20 mg sodium
	6 g carbohydrate
UHEP	3/4 Fat
	2 1/4 Vegetables & Fruit

Stir-Fried Broccoli with Cashews

Every so often a culinary inspiration comes floating down from the Food Gods. This recipe is a case in point. There I was all alone in the kitchen chopping broccoli when all of a sudden out of the blue it hit me—cashews! I am so glad that I listen to my inner child cook, because this has become one of my house specialties.

Sauce
3/4 cup / 175 mL **chicken stock or lower-sodium chicken stock**
3 tbsp / 45 mL **oyster sauce**
2 tsp / 10 mL **chili garlic sauce**
1 1/2 tsp / 7 mL **cornstarch**

2 tsp / 10 mL **extra virgin olive oil**
1 **Vidalia onion**
4 cups / 1 L **broccoli florets**
1/2 cup / 125 mL **unsalted cashews**

1   Mix together the sauce ingredients and set aside.

2   Cut the onion into 1/4-in/0.6-cm diagonal slices.

4   Heat a nonstick frying pan or a wok. Add the oil, heat. Add the onion. Stir-fry for 30 seconds.

5   Add the broccoli and stir-fry for 2 to 4 minutes or until it's tender-crisp.

6   Add the sauce ingredients and stir until the sauce thickens. Add cashews. Serve.

Serves 4

WHERE DO I FIND?

1. Chili Garlic Sauce—you can find this spicy blend of garlic and chilis in the Asian section of your grocery store. Once you open it, store it in the fridge. It will last up to 1 year.

2. Oyster Sauce—in the same section! Same deal.

SERVING TIP

Tastes great over brown rice or whole-wheat pasta.

ONE SERVING	157 Calories
	5.6 g protein
	10.9 g fat
	3.0 g fiber
	287 mg sodium
	12 g carbohydrate
lower-sodium chicken stock	217 mg
UHEP	1/2 Fat
	2 1/4 Vegetables & Fruit
	1/2 Nuts

Brussels Sprouts, or "How Do I Get Them to Eat Those Things?"

SERVING TIP
If you really think that the Brussels sprouts will go over like a lead balloon, use broccoli instead, and try the next recipe.

Growing up I thought that Brussels sprouts were supposed to be cooked for at least 30 minutes. That's how my grandmother and mom cooked them. They were always grey blobs of mush that my parents and grandparents ate, but not me, nor my brother or sister. My mom cooked all the other vegetables so that they were edible, but Brussels sprouts—big loser.

It wasn't until I went to university that I discovered "tender-crisp" vegetables—veggies that were "just" cooked, full of flavor and color!

I am sure that most people who don't like Brussels sprouts have had a similar "bad sprout experience" and the memory of that has scarred them for life. Well, here are two recipes that might be able to change that. Give them a try.

Stir-Fried Brussels Sprouts and Carrots

Have you ever had stir-fried "sprouts?" Most people haven't. My partner, Scott, hates sprouts. This is the only way that he will eat them! Try them out on one of your sprout-challenged friends.

1 tbsp + 1 tsp / 20 mL **extra virgin olive oil**
2 cups / 500 mL **Brussels sprouts—15 large, 30 small cut in half**
2 **large carrots—chopped**
1 tbsp / 15 mL **minced ginger**
1/4 cup / 50 mL **chicken stock or lower-sodium chicken stock**

1   In a large frying pan, heat the oil.

2   Add the Brussels sprouts, carrots and ginger. Stir-fry till coated with the oil.

3   Add the chicken stock. Cover, reduce the heat to simmer, and cook for 5 minutes or until the veggies are just cooked.

4   Serve. Wait for the, "Hey these are good!"

Serves 4

ONE SERVING	76 Calories
	2.1 g protein
	4.6 g fat
	2.8 g fiber
	84 mg sodium
	8 g carbohydrate
lower-sodium chicken stock	61 mg sodium
UHEP	1 Fat
	2 Vegetables & Fruit

Brussels Sprouts (cont.)

Brussels Sprouts with Maple Syrup

For the sweet tooth in the family, these "Brussels" with maple syrup may be just the thing!

2 cups / 500 mL **Brussels sprouts—15 large—30 small**
1 tbsp / 15 mL **maple syrup**
1 tbsp / 15 mL **nonhydrogenated margarine**

1 Wash the sprouts and cut off the woody stems.

2 Put in a large pot and barely cover with water.

3 Bring to a gentle boil, cover and cook for 5 to 7 minutes or until tender. Take one out and taste it. Too hard? Cook a couple of minutes more.

4 Drain. Add the maple syrup and butter to the bright green Brussels sprouts.

5 Mix until coated and that's it! I'll say it again: some vegetables taste best when they haven't been done up too much or cooked to death!

Serves 4

STILL HATE BRUSSELS SPROUTS?
Okay, at least you tried.

STEAMING
If you prefer to steam them instead of boiling, it takes 8 to 10 minutes.

ONE SERVING	59 Calories
	1.5 g protein
	3.2 g fat
	1.7 g fiber
	31 mg sodium
	7 g carbohydrate
UHEP	3/4 Fat
	1 Vegetables & Fruit

Roasted Garlic Potatoes

COMPANY POTATOES
Add 1 tbsp/15 mL of chopped fresh rosemary to the olive oil and the potatoes. Then follow the recipe as is.

Here is my dream question on *Jeopardy*:
Me—*I'll take vegetable-storing questions for $1000, Alex.*
Alex Trebeck—*This potato loves to be stored in the fridge.*
Me—*What is—a new potato?*
Alex—*You are right and take the lead with $68,000!*
If you ever get to *Jeopardy* and get this answer right because of me, I would like a thank-you note at the very least. Yes, the only type of potato that likes being in the fridge is the new potato. Store them in a plastic bag for up to 1 week. Then either steam them or roast them.

20 **new baby potatoes**
1 tbsp + 1 tsp / 20 mL **extra virgin olive oil**
1 **lemon, juice of—in 2 portions**
salt—optional
freshly cracked pepper
8 **cloves garlic**

1 Preheat oven to 400°F/200°C.

2 Wash the potatoes and cut into quarters.

3 Toss the potatoes with the olive oil and 1/2 the lemon juice.

4 Line a 9 x 13-in/23 x 33-cm pan with parchment paper or foil. Dump in the potatoes.

5 Sprinkle on the salt and pepper, if using.

6 Put the potatoes in the oven and roast for 30–45 minutes.

7 Wrap the garlic in a piece of foil. Roast in the oven for 30 minutes or until soft.

8 Pop the roasted garlic out of its peel. Mix with the remaining lemon juice. Set aside.

9 When the potatoes are cooked, dump them into a large bowl. Toss with the garlic/lemon mixture. Serve.

Serves 4

ONE SERVING	
	147 Calories
	2.9 g protein
	4.8 g fat
	2.1 g fiber
	8 mg sodium
	25 g carbohydrate
UHEP	1 Fat
	2 1/2 Vegetables & Fruit

Grains

Wild and Brown Rice

BROWN RICE

Brown rice is the only whole-grain rice in the rice family. It is the entire grain with only the tough inedible outer husk removed. It comes in both short and long grain. If you want a stickier rice choose the short grain; if you are looking for a fluffier rice, then go with the long grain.

There is a parboiled type of brown rice available but it isn't a whole grain and therefore not as nutritious and without nearly as much of the fiber that the regular brown rice has. Don't use it.

Whole-grain brown rice does take longer to cook than any of the other rices, but its nutty texture and flavor are well worth the 45-minute wait.

When cooking brown rice make sure that you are using a heavy-bottomed pot with a tight-fitting lid. Always bring the rice to the boil, cover and reduce the heat to simmer. Time it according to the recipe and under no circumstances peek into the pot or worse still, mix it! These are big no-nos that will cause the rice to become gummy and taste like glue. Next time you are making a pot of brown rice, double it and store it in the fridge. It will keep for up to 3 days.

Here are three of my household standbys.

Whenever I serve this rice dish, people always want the recipe. When I tell them it's just wild rice, brown rice and chicken stock, they are stunned.

1/4 cup / 50 mL **wild rice**
3/4 cup / 175 mL **long-grain brown rice**
2 cups / 500 mL **chicken stock or lower-sodium chicken stock**

1 In a heavy pot mix the wild rice, brown rice and chicken stock.

2 Bring to a boil. Cover with a tight-fitting lid and reduce heat to simmer. Cook 45 to 50 minutes or until all the liquid has been absorbed.

3 Fluff with a fork. Remove from heat and let sit for 10 minutes. Serve. Hand out papers and pencils for the recipe giveaway.

Serves 6

ONE SERVING	113 Calories
	3.4 g protein
	0.8 g fat
	1.2 g fiber
	326 mg sodium
	23 g carbohydrate
lower-sodium chicken stock	202 mg
UHEP	1 Grains

9/10

Brown Rice with Dried Cranberries and Orange

If you happen to go a Cranberry Festival in October and get caught up in the frenzy of cranberry lust causing you to purchase a 20-lb/9-kg bag of cranberries, then you are going to love this recipe!

You can either freeze those cranberries or buy a food dehydrator and dry your own—that might be a bit Marthaesque, but it's your call. I personally froze the entire 20-lb/9-kg bag and bought Craisins at the grocery store for this recipe. I have vowed never to buy anything larger than my trunk again.

1 cup / 250 mL **long-grain brown rice**
2 cups / 500 mL **chicken stock or lower-sodium chicken stock**
1 **onion—minced**
1/2 cup / 125 mL **dried cranberries or Craisins** (see page 257)
1 **orange—zest of**

1 In a medium pot mix together the brown rice, chicken stock and onion. Bring to the boil. Cover with a tight-fitting lid. Reduce heat to simmer and cook for 40 minutes.

2 Add the dried cranberries. Cover and continue cooking for 5 minutes or until the rice is tender.

3 Remove from heat. Stir the rice gently. Add the orange zest and serve.

Serves 6

ONE SERVING	130 Calories
	3.3 g protein
	1.0 g fat
	1.8 g fiber
	327 mg sodium
	27 g carbohydrate
lower-sodium chicken stock	203 mg sodium
UHEP	1 Grains
	1/4 Vegetables & Fruit

SO WHAT THE HECK IS A REALLY GOOD PARMESAN?

Well, it's not the stuff that comes out of a can! My favorite is Parmigiano-Reggiano, which comes from, you guessed it, Italy! It has a sharp, rich flavor that makes a little go a long way. You buy this at the deli counter or the cheese counter in most grocery stores. It comes as a block of cheese and you grate as you need it.

SO WHAT THE HECK DOES KALE LOOK LIKE ANYWAY?

Well it's in the produce section and it's usually tucked away with the other not-so-popular vegetables! You won't find it beside the carrots! It has very dark green frilly leaves and is usually sold in bunches. It's a member of the cabbage family with a much milder taste than its stronger-tasting family members. Whenever I serve it to my son's friends he always tells them that it doesn't taste like anything! What he means is that, with its intense green color you would think that it would have a very intense flavor. Well, wrong! It has a very mild flavor that is surprisingly deli-cious. Buy the smaller frilly leaves—they are more tender as well. Always remove the leaves from the stalk before cooking. The stalk tends to have a bitter flavor even though the leaves don't.

ONE SERVING	203 Calories
	7.5 g protein
	2.8 g fat
	4.9 g fiber
	587 mg sodium
	39 g carbohydrate
lower-sodium chicken stock	401 mg
UHEP	1 3/4 Vegetables & Fruit
	1 Grains

Short-Grain Brown Rice Risotto with Kale and Squash

Kid-Approved

All you risotto lovers are going to take one look at this recipe and say no way! There isn't a hope in h— that this is going to be creamy and delicious like a real risotto. Even when you ignore the gobs of fat in a real risotto, arborio rice still has no redeeming nutritional qualities, but brown rice, squash and kale do!

3 cups / 750 mL **butternut squash—about 1/2 of a medium butternut squash**
3 cups / 750 mL **chicken stock or lower-sodium chicken stock**
1 **medium onion—diced**
4 **cloves garlic—minced**
1 cup / 250 mL **short-grain brown rice**
4 cups / 1 L **kale—stems removed and discarded—leaves chopped**
1/4 cup / 50 mL **Parmesan—Reggiano**

1   Peel the squash and then cut it into 1-in/2.5-cm cubes. (Use the end without the seeds, it's easier to chop up!) Save the other end to roast in the oven another day.

2   In a medium-sized heavy-bottomed pot, mix together the chicken stock, onion, garlic, brown rice and squash. Bring to the boil. Stir, cover and reduce the heat to low. Simmer for 40 minutes. Set your timer, just in case you happen to forget about what you are cooking!

3   Cut the stalk from the kale leaves and then chop the leaves into small pieces. Discard stalks.

4   When the timer goes off, add the chopped kale. Stir in. This will look impossible, but be tenacious, it will stir in.

5   Simmer for 10 more minutes, stirring occasionally.

6   Sprinkle each serving with Parmesan.

Serves 6

Three Favorite Bulgar Recipes

What an education you are getting reading and cooking through this book! Here's another new food—bulgar. So what is it anyway? Bulgar is wheat kernels that have been steamed, dried and crushed! It only takes 20 minutes to cook and is a great alternative to brown rice. It has a tender, chewy texture and is a great side dish for any of the salmon or chicken recipes in this book.

I have included three of my favorite recipes.

Bulgar Pilaf

If you've never had bulgar this is the beginner recipe! It's easy, flavorful and fast to make.

1 tbsp + 1 tsp / 20 mL **extra virgin olive oil**
1 **onion—diced**
6 **mushrooms—sliced thinly**
2 **cloves garlic—minced**
1 cup / 250 mL **bulgar**
2 cups / 500 mL **chicken stock or lower-sodium chicken stock**

1   Heat a medium pot. Add the oil.

2   Sauté the onion and mushrooms until the mushrooms begin to brown.

3   Add the garlic and bulgar. Stir till coated.

4   Add chicken stock and bring to a boil. Cover, reduce to simmer and cook for 20 minutes.

Serves 6

ONE SERVING	123 Calories
	4.3 g protein
	3.6 g fat
	4.7 g fiber
	330 mg sodium
	20 g carbohydrate
lower-sodium chicken stock	206 mg sodium
UHEP	3/4 Fat
	1 Grains

Orange Bulgar

This would be the second bulgar dish you might like to try. The flavor from the orange juice isn't overpowering and this goes really well with Baked Salmon with Fresh Citrus on page 214 or Company's Comin' Salmon on page 215.

1 cup / 250 mL **water**
1 cup / 250 mL **orange juice**
1 cup / 250 mL **bulgar**

1   In a medium saucepan bring the water and orange juice to the boil.

2   Add the bulgar. Cover with a lid, reduce the heat to simmer.

3   Simmer for 15 minutes. Remove from the heat. Let sit 5 minutes. Fluff with a fork and serve.

Serves 6

ONE SERVING	100 Calories
	3.2 g protein
	0.3 g fat
	4.3 g fiber
	5 mg sodium
	22 g carbohydrate
UHEP	1/4 Vegetables & Fruit
	1 Grains

Three Favorite Bulgar Recipes (cont.)

Spicy Bulgar Pilaf

For the real bulgar lover or a foodie risk-taker! Here is a
more challenging recipe—in flavor only. It's still easy
and fast to make, but has a definite spicy note to it.

1 tbsp + 1 tsp / 20 mL **extra virgin olive oil**
1 **sweet onion—Vidalia—diced**
1 **green pepper—chopped coarsely**
1/2 **red pepper—chopped coarsely**
1 **stalk celery—chopped coarsely**
2 **cloves garlic—minced**
1 tsp / 5 mL **thyme**
1/4 tsp / 1 mL **red pepper flakes**
1 cup / 250 mL **bulgar**
2 cups / 500 mL **chicken stock or lower-sodium chicken stock**

1   Heat a medium pot. Add the oil.

2   Sauté the onion, green and red peppers, celery and garlic
    till the onion is translucent.

3   Add the thyme, red pepper flakes and bulgar. Stir till
    coated.

4   Pour in the chicken stock and bring to a boil. Cover,
    reduce to simmer and cook for 20 minutes.

Serves 6

ONE SERVING	132 Calories
	4.2 g protein
	3.6 g fat
	5.4 g fiber
	335 mg sodium
	23 g carbohydrate
lower-sodium chicken stock	211 mg sodium
UHEP	3/4 Fat
	1/2 Vegetables & Fruit
	1 Grains

Quinoa Pilaf

WHERE THE HECK DO I FIND QUINOA?

If your grocery store has a health food section, it's probably there, in with the other grains. If not, most health food stores carry it.

This ancient grain was eaten by the Incas centuries ago. They called quinoa (pronounced keen-wah) the "mother grain" and it has been called the "supergrain of the future."

Quinoa contains more protein than any other grain and is a nutrition powerhouse. It has a very unique shape and is very bitter if it isn't rinsed thoroughly. It has a really odd shape when cooked—looks like mini spirals, so don't expect it to look like rice! Just warning you.

Quinoa alone has a very mild flavor and looks fairly boring. But when you add the curry and the turmeric it goes from boring and blah to fantastic and flavorful!

1 tbsp + 1 tsp / 20 mL **extra virgin olive oil**
1 **onion—chopped**
1 cup / 250 mL **quinoa**
1 tsp / 5 mL **turmeric**
1/2 tsp / 2 mL **curry powder**
1/2 tsp / 2 mL **allspice**
2 cups / 500 mL **vegetable stock or lower-sodium chicken stock**

1   In a medium pot heat the olive oil. Add the onion and sauté for 1 minute.

2   Rinse the quinoa in a tight-meshed strainer. It will fall through the holes in a colander. Rinse well.

3   Add the quinoa to the onion. Add the turmeric, curry powder, allspice and vegetable stock.

4   Bring to the boil. Cover with a tight-fitting lid. Reduce heat to simmer and cook for 20 minutes.

Serves 8

ONE SERVING	113 Calories
vegetable stock	3.1 g protein
	3.7 g fat
	1.7 g fiber
	182 mg sodium
	18 g carbohydrate
lower-sodium chicken stock	155 mg sodium
regular chicken stock	248 mg sodium
UHEP	1 Grains

Barley Risotto

In my humble culinary opinion, risotto is the utimate
Italian comfort food. Its creamy consistency and rich flavors
of garlic, chicken stock and Parmesan cheese are incredibly
delicious and soothing all at the same time. On a cold
winter night, not many things beat a great dish of risotto.
Well, okay, I can think of a couple things . . .

This version uses the whole-grain pearl barley, which
lends itself to a creamy texture. Enjoy!

1 tbsp + 1 tsp / 20 mL **extra virgin olive oil**
2 **onions—diced**
2 **portabello mushrooms—chopped coarsely**
3 **cloves garlic—minced**
3/4 cup / 175 mL **pearl barley**
2 1/2 cups / 625 mL **chicken stock or lower-sodium chicken stock**
1/4 cup / 50 mL **Parmesan—Reggiano** (see page 181)

1   Heat a medium saucepan, add the olive oil and sauté the
    onions.

2   Add the mushrooms and the garlic and continue
    sautéing for 1 minute.

3   Add the pearl barley and the chicken stock. Stir. Bring to
    the boil. Reduce the heat to simmer, cover with a tightly
    fitting lid and simmer for 50 minutes. Stir occasionally. If
    it looks dry add 1/4 cup/50 mL water.

4   Remove from heat, gently stir in the Parmesan and serve.

    Serves 8

ONE SERVING	113 Calories
	3.9 g protein
	3.5 g fat
	0.6 g fiber
	364 mg sodium
	17 g carbohydrate
lower-sodium chicken stock	248 mg sodium
UHEP	1/2 Fat
	1/4 Vegetables & Fruit
	1/2 Grains

Pasta

6/10 – leave out broccoli

Asian Noodle Salad

This is a great summer salad that you can make early on in the day or even the night before. It blends the flavors of peanuts, chili peppers, cabbage and whole-wheat spaghetti to give you an Asian flair with just a little bit of spice.

1 cup / 250 mL **whole-wheat spaghetti**
4 cups / approx. 1 L **shredded red cabbage**
1 **large carrot**
1 **red pepper**
4 cups / 1 L **broccoli florets**

Dressing
1/4 cup / 50 mL **crunchy peanut butter**
2 tbsp / 25 mL **rice vinegar**
2 tbsp / 25 mL **water**
2 tbsp / 25 mL **sodium-reduced soy sauce**
2 tbsp / 25 **mL honey**
1 tbsp / 15 mL **chili garlic sauce** (see page 174)
1 **lime—juice of**

Toppings
1/4 cup / 50 mL **peanuts**
1 cup / 250 mL **chopped fresh cilantro** optional, but it really does give it an authentic Asian flavor
1 **green onion—chopped** optional

1   Put water on to boil. Measure out 1 cup/250 mL dry whole-wheat spaghetti. That is equal to about 1 big handful. You want enough cooked pasta to equal 2 cups/500 mL. When the water comes to the boil, break the spaghetti in half and cook until just done, about 8 minutes.

WHERE DO I FIND RICE VINEGAR?
You can find this mild-tasting vinegar along with all the other vinegars. If for some reason you can't find it, use cider vinegar instead.

WHAT KIND OF PEANUT BUTTER SHOULD I USE?
I like the "nothing but peanuts" kind. Yes, it is messy compared to the other types of peanut butter, but I don't mind mixing it up before I store it in the fridge. I like the way it tastes. So for my taste buds I pick the "unadulterated" peanut butter. You can buy it at your grocery store where all the other types of peanut butter are sold, or at a health food store.

Not everyone likes this kind of peanut butter. The bottom line is, buy the kind that you will eat.

SERVING TIP

If you like, parboil the broccoli before adding to the rest of the ingredients.

KID-FRIENDLY TIP

If your kids aren't into spicy, omit the chili garlic sauce. At serving time, dish theirs out, then add the chili garlic sauce to the rest. Toss well. Serve to the adults.

My son has been eating spicy foods since he was seven, so don't give up. Offer them some of the spicy version. One day they may just surprise you and ask for it!

2 Meanwhile shred the cabbage, grate the carrot and chop the red pepper. Cut the broccoli florets from the stacks. Cut the florets into small pieces. The pieces should be small enough to pop into your mouth without looking rude!

3 Put all the veggies into a large bowl. Toss and set aside.

4 For the dressing, measure out the peanut butter, rice vinegar, water, soy sauce, honey, chili garlic sauce and lime juice into a bowl and whisk till blended.

5 Pour the dressing over the veggies.

6 By this time the spaghetti should be cooked. Drain. Add to the veggies and toss until everything is well-coated with the dressing.

7 Refrigerate till well chilled, either 3 hours or up to overnight.

8 At serving time, divide the salad equally among four plates and sprinkle each serving with peanuts. If you decided to go with the Asian flavors sprinkle each with the cilantro and green onion.

Serves 4

ONE SERVING	350 calories
	14.4 g protein
	14.5 g fat
	9.0 g fiber
	516 mg sodium
	46 g carbohydrate
UHEP	4 Vegetables & Fruit
	1 Grains
	1 Nuts

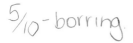
5/10 - borring

Rotini with Plum Tomatoes and Lentils

My sister, Kathleen, doesn't like lentils. As a matter of fact, she hates them! Last year she came for a visit from Vancouver. She arrived at 9 p.m., starving. The only thing that I had in the fridge was my "Rotini with Plum Tomatoes and Lentil" dish. I heated it up. She took one look them and said, "I'm not eating those things, Mair, you know I hate them!" I convinced her that they were really very good, so reluctantly she gave them a taste, and to her surprise, but not mine, she loved them! She even had a second helping! The true test that a recipe is great.

1 tbsp + 1 tsp / 20 mL **extra virgin olive oil**
1 **onion—diced**
1 **clove garlic—minced**
1/2 cup / 125 mL **roasted red pepper—chopped** (see page 193)
1 28 fl oz / 796 mL can **plum tomatoes**
1 19 fl oz/540 mL can **lentils—drained and rinsed**
2 tbsp / 25 mL **tomato paste**
1 tsp / 5 mL **Worcestershire sauce**
1 tsp / 5 mL **basil**
1/4 tsp / 1 mL **red pepper flakes**
1 1/2 cups / 375 mL **uncooked whole-wheat rotini**
2 tbsp / 25 mL **Parmesan** (see page 181)

1 Put a large pot of water on to boil.

2 Heat a large skillet. Add the olive oil. Sauté the onions for 3 minutes stirring occasionally.

3 Add the garlic and sauté for 1 minute, stirring constantly. (Remember—burnt garlic is awful!)

4 And the roasted red pepper and the tomatoes. Mash the tomatoes with a fork.

5 Add the lentils, tomato paste, Worcestershire sauce, basil and red pepper flakes. Bring to a boil. Cover and reduce heat to simmer. Cook for 10 minutes, stirring occasionally.

6 Meanwhile back to that pot of water! When it comes to a boil add the rotini. Stir. Cook until al dente—about 10 minutes.

7 When the pasta is cooked, drain. Add to the tomato-lentil mixture. Stir well. Let simmer 5 minutes.

8 Serve with Parmesan on each serving.

Serves 4

QUICK DINNER TIP

Steam broccoli after you add the pasta to the lentil mixture. The broccoli will be cooked at the same time that the lentils are ready!

BOILING PASTA

Use lots of water to boil pasta and don't add oil! Bring the water to the boil, add the pasta, give it a stir to prevent it from sticking to the bottom of the pot. Bring it back to the boil and then begin timing. When it's cooked, drain, but never rinse! Rinsing does two bad things. One, it rinses off nutrients and two, it rinses off the starch that helps the sauce stick to it.

AL DENTE?

It literally means "to the tooth." Which, translated to cookery terms, means "don't cook the hell out of it!" Pasta should have some kind of texture. A lot of people cook it till it's mushy, which is a huge no-no. Read the package and follow the directions.

ONE SERVING	356 Calories
	17.2 g protein
	7.5 g fat
	10.6 g fiber
	802 mg sodium
	57 g carbohydrate
UHEP	1 Beans
	1 Fat
	2 Vegetables & Fruit
	1 1/2 Grains

Pasta Primavera

"Primavera" means "spring" in Italian—but I serve this dish as long as I can get great-tasting asparagus! This recipe is an Italian stir-fry that you toss with the cooked pasta and then sprinkle with Parmesan cheese. Simple ingredients to make a terrific dinner!

8 **stalks asparagus**
2 cups / 500 mL **kale** (see page 181)
2 cups / 500 mL **cherry or grape tomatoes**
1 cups / 375 mL **dry whole-wheat penne**
2 tsp / 10 mL **extra virgin olive oil**
2 cups / 500 mL **broccoli florets**
1 **onion**
4 **cloves garlic—minced**
1 cup / 250 mL **vegetable stock or lower-sodium chicken stock**
2 tbsp / 25 mL **balsamic vinegar**
1/4 cup / 50 mL **Parmesan** (see page 181)
1 cup / 250 mL **basil leaves—chopped**
freshly cracked pepper to taste

1 Put a large pot of water on to boil.

2 Remove woody ends from the asparagus, chop remaining asparagus stalk into 3 pieces.

3 Remove the kale from the stalk and chop the leaves coarsely. Discard stalks.

4 Cut the tomatoes in halves.

5 Put the pasta on to cook.

6 Heat a large frying pan. Add the oil. Stir-fry the broccoli and the onion. Add the asparagus, kale, tomatoes and garlic. Stir-fry.

7 Add the stock and balsamic vinegar. Cover and simmer for 2 to 3 minutes or until the vegetables are tender-crisp.

8 Add the basil.

9 Drain the cooked pasta and toss in with the veggies.

10 Serve with Parmesan cheese.

Serves 4

ONE SERVING	248 Calories
	10.6 g protein
vegetable stock	5.8 g fat
	6.9 g fiber
	329 mg sodium
	41 g carbohydrate
lower-sodium chicken stock	302 mg sodium
regular chicken stock	396 mg sodium
UHEP	1/2 Fat
	3 Vegetables & Fruit
	1 1/2 Grains
	1/4 Milk

Rotini with Feta and Tomatoes

This recipe appeared in my first cookbook *Lick the Spoon!* in 1998. I updated the recipe a couple of years ago, and quite frankly I like this version better!

It's a noncooked sauce! So chop up the tomatoes, mince up the onion and open the vino while the pasta is cooking!

1 1/2 cups / 375 mL **dry whole-wheat rotini**
4 **large tomatoes—chopped into bite-sized pieces**
1/3 cup / 75 mL **minced red onion**
8 **olives—pitted**
4 oz / 1 cup/ 250 mL / 110 g **light feta—crumbled**
2 tbsp / 25 mL **balsamic vinegar**

1   Put a large pot of water on to boil. Add the whole-wheat rotini and cook for 9 to 10 minutes or until tender. Open up a bottle of red wine. Let breathe. Sip while prepping the veggies!

2   Combine the tomatoes, minced red onion, pitted olives, crumbled feta cheese and the balsamic vinegar.

3   When the pasta is cooked, drain and pour over tomato mixture.

4   Toss. Crack on some fresh pepper and serve.

Serves 4

ONE SERVING	276 Calories
	6.0 g protein
	8.0 g fat
	4.4 g fiber
	93 mg sodium
	35 g carbohydrate
UHEP	2 Vegetables & Fruit
	1 1/2 Grains
	1/2 Milk

Mairlyn's Amazing Tomato Sauce

KID-FRIENDLY TIP

Garlic Alert! If you have really young children, they may find the garlic too intense. The kids who have eaten this and loved it were usually over 5 years old! If you feel that your child will not like the garlic, feel free to downgrade to 4 cloves.

ROASTED RED PEPPERS: HOW TO MAKE THEM. YOUR PICK!

1. Go to the grocery store and buy a bottle of roasted red peppers in a wine vinegar broth. That may sound hard to find but surprisingly it isn't! I usually buy Krinos, a product from Greece. The peppers are packed whole in a wine vinegar broth, not oil. I just slice them in half and use them in the recipe.

OR

2. Wash and dry 3 very ripe red peppers. Cut them in half and remove the seeds. Roast in a 400°F/200°C oven till the skins are blackened. Let cool. Remove the blackened skins and use in the recipe.

Make this sauce once and end up with two different dinners for a family of four. The first night serve it on whole-wheat pasta with a sprinkle of a really good Parmesan. Each serving is 3/4 cup/175 mL sauce over 1 1/2 cups/375 mL pasta. Then the next night or two nights later, use the remaining sauce for the lasagna recipe on the next page. Or double the recipe and freeze it in 3 cup/750 mL portions. A great freezeable!

2 tbsp / 25 mL	**extra virgin olive oil**
1	**large onion—diced**
8	**cloves garlic—minced**
2 28-fl oz / 796-mL cans	**plum tomatoes**
3	**whole roasted red peppers—chopped coarsely** (see sidebar)
2 tbsp / 25 mL	**chopped fresh basil**

1   Heat a large pot. Add the oil. Sauté the onion till golden, about 5 minutes.

2   Add the garlic, stir till coated in the oil. Don't let it burn or the sauce will be ruined!

3   Add the plum tomatoes. Mash with a potato masher. Bring to the boil.

4   Add the chopped roasted red peppers. Mash again. Simmer for 25 minutes or until the sauce starts getting thicker.

5   Add the fresh basil. Remove from the heat. Serve over cooked whole-wheat pasta.

Serves 8. Makes 6 cups/1.5 L.

ONE SERVING tomato sauce	106 Calories 2.8 g protein 4.2 g fat 5.2 g fiber 440 mg sodium 15 g carbohydrate
UHEP	1 Fat 1 Vegetables & Fruit
ONE SERVING tomato sauce with pasta	425 Calories 13.8 g protein 6.2 g fat 10.2 g fiber 442 mg sodium 79 g carbohydrate
UHEP	1 Fat 1 Vegetables & Fruit 3 Grains

7/10

Spinach Lasagna

A really easy lasagna to whip up, especially if you have the sauce already made! I serve this with either steamed broccoli or a side salad and whole wheat rolls.

9 **whole-wheat lasagna noodles**
1 10-oz / 284-g pkg. **spinach**
1 18-oz / 500-mL **container light ricotta**
1 **egg**
1/2 cup / 125 mL **really good Parmesan** (see page 181)
3 cups / 750 mL **Tomato Sauce** (see page 193)
1/3 cup / 175 mL **grated skim milk mozzarella**

1 Preheat the oven to 350°F/175°C.

2 Bring a large pot of water to the boil. Add the whole-wheat noodles and cook for 10 minutes or until al dente.

3 Meanwhile wash the spinach and steam till just limp, approx. 2 to 3 minutes. Drain. Let sit in the colander till cooled. Squeeze out excess water. Chop coarsely. Set aside.

4 Mix together the ricotta, egg and Parmesan. Set aside.

5 Drain the noodles.

6 Now begin the layering—spread about 2 tbsp/25 mL of the tomato sauce in the bottom of a 9 x 13-in/23 x 33-cm pan. Lay 3 noodles on top. Spoon 1 cup/250 mL of the sauce on top. Spoon 1/3 of the cheese mixture on top. Sprinkle with 1/4 cup/50 mL of the mozzarella.

7 Lay on 3 noodles. Spoon on 1 cup/250 mL of the sauce. Top with the next third of the cheese mixture. Sprinkle with 1/4 cup/50 mL of the mozzarella.

8 Lay on the last 3 noodles. Spoon on the last of the tomato sauce. Spoon on the last of the cheese mixture. Spoon on the chopped spinach. Sprinkle with the last of the mozzarella.

9 Bake for 40 minutes. Remove from the oven and let "rest" for 10 minutes. This will help prevent the dreaded "lasagna mush mess" that occurs when it's cut right after coming out of the oven. Those 10 minutes really are worth the wait.

Serves 8

KID-FRIENDLY TIP
They don't like spinach? Chop it up and add it to the tomato sauce layer. Tell them it's basil. (Once in a while it's okay to tell culinary white lies.)

ONE SERVING	433 Calories
	25.5 g protein
	16.0 g fat
	7.3 g fiber
	699 mg sodium
	47 g carbohydrate
UHEP	1/2 Fat
	2 Vegetables & Fruit
	2 Grains
	1 Milk

Tuna Pasta Salad

Back in the '60s when I was a kid, my friend's mom used to make a great tuna pasta salad. It was loaded with celery, green onions, tuna and about 4 cups/1 L of mayo. We would pick out the celery and the onions and just eat the tuna, pasta and mayo! It was sooo good, sooo white-looking and sooo loaded with fat! Too much fat.

What I needed to do was to create a recipe without all that mayo. Well, getting rid of most of the mayo got rid of most of the flavor. So I tried a totally different approach. I got rid of all of it and created a whole new taste sensation from scratch. Sort of like "out with the old, in with the new"—a taste divorce. Here's the new one.

1 1/2 cups / 375 mL **dry whole-wheat rotini**

2 6-oz / 170-g cans **lower-sodium tuna—well drained and cut into small chunks**

2 cups / 500 mL **grape or cherry tomatoes—cut into quarters**

1/2 cup / 125 mL **diced red onion**

1 **red pepper—diced**

1/3 / 75 mL cup **basil**

1/4 cup / 50 mL **parsley—chopped**

12 **spicy black olives—pitted—and cut into halves**

6 **green olives—pitted—chopped**

Dressing

4 **sundried tomatoes**

1 **roasted red pepper** (see page 193)

1/2 cup / 125 mL **loosely packed basil**

1/3 cup / 75 mL **red wine vinegar**

4 **cloves garlic**

2 tsp / 10 mL **extra virgin olive oil**

1   Put a large pot of water on to boil. Add the whole-wheat rotini and cook for 9 to 10 minutes or until tender.

2   In a large bowl mix together the tuna, tomatoes, red onion, red pepper, basil, parsley and black and green olives. Set aside.

3   In the food processor or blender purée the dressing ingredients. Pour over the tuna mixture.

4   Drain the pasta. Add to the tuna mixture. Mix well. Store covered in the fridge for up to 3 days.

Serves 4. Makes 8 cups/2 L.

ONE SERVING	307 Calories
	23.2 g protein
	6.7 g fat
	5.9 g fiber
	210 mg sodium
	42 g carbohydrate
UHEP	1 Fat
	1 Fish
	1 1/2 Vegetables & Fruit
	1 1/2 Grains

Spicy Turkey Pasta Sauce

I have really mixed feelings about ground turkey. (Spoken like a true foodie!) I like the leanness that it offers a recipe, but I don't like its blah flavor. Enter Mairlyn's Spicy Turkey Pasta Sauce! This tried and true recipe has tons of flavor, so don't be surprised that it calls for 6 cloves of garlic and 2 tbsp/25 mL of dried basil! They really "tune" this recipe right up, taking out the blah and adding a baboom!

1 tbsp / 15 mL **extra virgin olive oil**
2 **onions**
1 1/4 lb / 560 g **extra lean ground turkey**
6 **cloves garlic**
2 tbsp / 25 mL **dried basil**
1 tsp / 5 mL **oregano**
1/4 tsp / 1 mL **thyme**
2 28-fl oz / 796-mL cans **plum tomatoes**
2 5 1/2-fl oz / 156-mL cans **tomato paste**
1 cup / 250 mL **red wine**
2 tsp / 10 mL **honey**
2 tsp / 10 mL **Worcestershire sauce**
1/4 tsp / 1 mL **black pepper**
1/4 tsp / 1 mL **cayenne—optional**

1 In a large covered pot heat the olive oil and sauté the onion for 2 minutes.

2 Add the ground turkey and brown.

3 Add the garlic, basil, oregano, thyme, plum tomatoes, tomato paste, red wine, honey, Worcestershire sauce, black pepper and cayenne. (In other words, everything else in the recipe!)

4 Stir well. Bring to the boil. Reduce heat, cover and simmer for 20 minutes.

5 Serve over 1 cup/250 mL of cooked spaghetti. Sprinkle with Parmesan if desired.

Serves 8. Makes 8 cups/2 L.

ONE SERVING	176 Calories
	9.5 g protein
	5.0 g fat
	6.4 g fiber
	815 mg sodium
	23 g carbohydrate
UHEP	1/4 Fat
	1 Vegetables & Fruit
	1 Meat
ONE SERVING with 1 cup/ 250mL cooked whole-wheat spaghetti	389 Calories
	16.8 g protein
	6.3 g fat
	9.8 g fiber
	816 mg sodium
	66 g carbohydrate
UHEP	1/4 Fat
	1 Vegetables & Fruit
	2 Grains
	1 Meat

Poultry

Chicken with Mango and Apricots

This is easy enough to make any night of the week! But it's also elegant enough to serve to someone you would like to impress the socks off.

Of all the recipes that I created for our book, this is Liz's favorite and it has now become her house speciality.

14 oz / 400 g **boneless skinless chicken breasts—cut into 4 equal pieces**

Sauce
1 14 oz / 398 mL can **apricots—drained (reserve 1/3 cup/75 mL of the liquid)**
3 tbsp / 45 mL **frozen orange juice concentrate**
1/3 cup / 75 mL **mango chutney**
1 tbsp / 15 mL **sodium-reduced soy sauce**
1 **large very ripe mango**

1   Preheat the oven to 425°F/220°C.

2   Line an 8 x 8-in/20 x 20-cm pan with parchment paper or foil. Lay the chicken on top.

3   Drain the apricots making sure to reserve 1/3 cup/75 mL of the liquid. Set the apricots aside. Mix the reserved liquid together with the orange juice concentrate, mango chutney and soy sauce. Pour over the chicken. Bake in the oven for 20 to 25 minutes or until done (when juice from chicken runs clear).

4   While the chicken is baking, cut and peel the mango. See page 205. Cut it into 1-in/2.5-cm slices. Set aside, along with the apricots.

5   When the chicken is cooked, pour the liquid off into a frying pan. Leave the chicken in the pan and cover. Turn the heat onto high and add the apricots and mango. Bring to a boil and leave to reduce for about 5 minutes until slightly thickened. Pour over the chicken. Serve.

Serves 4

CAN'T FIND CANNED APRICOTS?
Use fresh ones and add 1/3 cup/75 mL of apricot nectar that you find in the juice aisle. It is sold in tetra pak packaging and is usually with the "drink boxes."

WHAT IS FROZEN ORANGE JUICE CONCENTRATE AND WHERE DO I FIND IT?
It is the frozen juice that you find in the frozen juice aisle. You knew that (see page 165).

WHAT IS A VERY RIPE MANGO?
Mangoes are in season from May to September. Look for heavy ones that have a skin that is golden yellow with red mottling. This will be a deliciously ripe mango loaded with flavor and nutrition. Keep a ripened mango in the fridge for up to 4 days. To ripen a green mango, store it in a paper bag on the counter till the skin turns golden yellow.

SERVING TIP
This goes really well with brown rice or bulgar. Also, when the sauce is reducing it's a great time to put on your veggies. A quick, easy dinner!

ONE SERVING	331 Calories
	32.3 g protein
	3.7 g fat
	0.6 g fiber
	547 mg sodium
	40 g carbohydrate
UHEP	1 Vegetables & Fruit
	1 Meat

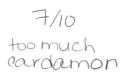

*7/10
too much
cardamon*

Chicken Biryani

Kid-Approved

SERVING TIP
Goes well with steamed broccoli or peas.

I have always loved international foods. I'm not a registered therapist, but in my layman's opinion it probably has something to do with being raised by British parents —they cooked the living daylights out of most foods. See Brussel Sprouts on page 175 for further details.

International foods, on the other hand, had flavors I had never experienced before. They did more than wake up my taste buds, they hit them over the head. This Chicken Biryani dish was one of the first international foods I ever ate. It is a milder version of an authentic biryani, but one that is still full of flavor and Indian spices.

1 tbsp + 1 tsp / 20 mL **extra virgin olive oil**
1 **medium onion—diced**
1/2 tsp / 2 mL **ground cumin**
1/2 tsp / 2 mL **ground cardamom**
1/2 tsp / 2 mL **pepper**
1/4 tsp / 1 mL **cloves**
1/2 tsp / 2 mL **cinnamon**
1 tsp / 5 mL **minced fresh ginger**
1 **large clove garlic**
14 oz / 400 g **skinless boneless chicken breasts—cut into bite-size pieces**
1 cup / 250 mL **1% yogurt**
1 1/4 cups / 300 mL **vegetable stock or lower-sodium chicken stock**
1 cup / 250 mL **bulgar**

1   Heat a large non-stick pan. Add the oil and sauté the onion for 1 minute.

2   Add the cumin, cardamom, pepper, cloves, cinnamon, ginger and garlic. Stir constantly. Savor the aromas.

3   Add the chicken and sauté till the outside of it is no longer pink.

4   Add the yogurt, stock, and bulgar. Stir till combined. Bring to the boil. Cover with a lid and reduce the heat to simmer. Cook for 20 minutes. Check to see that the chicken is cooked. Serve.

Serves 4

ONE SERVING	
	416 Calories
	37.7 g protein
vegetable stock	9.2 g fat
	1.9 g fiber
	594 mg sodium
	44 g carbohydrate
lower-sodium chicken stock	561 mg sodium
regular chicken stock	677 mg sodium
UHEP	1 Fat
	1 1/2 Grains
	1 Meat
	1/4 Milk

Chicken Tarragon

I grow tarragon. I planted it several years ago and have been trying to reclaim my garden ever since. If you ever want a great backdrop to your garden, go with tarragon. It looks great and you can eat it as well.

14 oz / 400 g skinless boneless chicken breasts—cut into 4 equal pieces

Sauce
1/2 cup / 125 mL **white wine**
1 cup / 250 mL **chicken stock or lower-sodium chicken stock**
3 tbsp / 45 mL **grainy Dijon mustard**
3 **cloves garlic—minced**
2 **shallots—minced**
1 tbsp / 15 mL **tarragon—chopped**
1/4 cup / 50 mL **2% evaporated milk**

1   Preheat the oven to 425°F/220°C.

2   Line an 8 x 8-in/20 x 20-cm pan with parchment paper or foil. Lay the chicken on top.

3   In a medium bowl mix together the white wine, chicken stock, grainy mustard, garlic and shallots. Pour over the chicken. This will cover it completely—you are going to be oven-poaching!

4   Oven-poach for 20 to 25 minutes.

5   When the chicken is cooked, pour off the liquid into a frying pan. Leave the chicken in the pan and cover. Bring the liquid to a boil and leave it to reduce for about 5 minutes until slightly thickened. Add the evaporated milk. Stir in. Add the tarragon. Heat through and pour this amazing sauce over the chicken!

Serves 4

WHAT IS GRAINY MUSTARD AND WHERE DO I FIND IT?

It is Dijon mustard with the mustard seeds still whole. It has a wonderfully intense mustard flavor. I use it a lot, so make sure you keep it in the fridge. You can find this terrific mustard with other types of mustard or sometimes in the gourmet section.

WHAT IS EVAPORATED 2% MILK AND WHERE DO I FIND IT?

It is usually beside the coffee and the tea in most grocery stores, with all the other canned milks. This is like regular canned milk, with less fat and without the awful tin taste! It is a great substitute for cream in most recipes and is terrific in this dish, if I do say so myself.

ONE SERVING	234 Calories
	34.3 g protein
	5.2 g fat
	0.6 g fiber
	564 mg sodium
	6 g carbohydrate
lower-sodium chicken stock	471 mg sodium
UHEP	1 Meat

Sundried Tomato Pesto with Chicken and Rotini

WHAT THE HECK ARE SUNDRIED TOMATOES AND WHERE DO I FIND THEM?

They are tomatoes that were supposedly dried in the sun! Go figure. They are packed in a number of different ways. I prefer the ones packed in olive oil, extra virgin if you can find it. Look in the section that carries the pickles and olives.

One of my favorite culinary memoirs is *Under the Tuscan Sun* by Frances Mayes, who bought a villa in Tuscany and spends her summers there. She describes the wonderful smells of fresh basil wafting in from her kitchen garden. I've always grown basil in big clay pots on the back stairs. Every time I go out with my kitchen scissors to snip the latest crop, I think of Frances under her Tuscan sun, and know that she too is enjoying the deliciously fragrant smells of her fresh basil.

2 cups / 500 mL **whole-wheat rotini**
14 oz / 400 g **skinless boneless chicken**

Topping
12 **sundried tomatoes—packed in olive oil**
6 **cloves garlic**
1/3 cup / 75 mL **vegetable broth or lower-sodium chicken stock**
1/2 cup /125 mL **fresh basil**
1 cup / 250 mL **2% evaporated milk**

1   Put a large pot of water on to boil. When boiling, add the rotini and cook for 9 to 10 minutes.

2   Lay the tomatoes on a paper towel to absorb some of the olive oil. When most of the oil has been absorbed chop the tomatoes coarsely.

3   In a food processor or a blender purée the garlic and broth.

4   Add the tomatoes and basil and pulse till combined. Set aside.

5   Slice the chicken into 1/4-in/0.6-cm slices.

6   Heat a large nonstick frying pan. Add the chicken and stir-fry till cooked. Remove from pan, add the tomato mixture and cook, stirring constantly for 1 minute.

7   Add the evaporated milk. Bring to the boil. Add the chicken and heat through. Remove from heat. Drain the cooked pasta and add to the chicken mixture. Serve.

Serves 4

ONE SERVING	442 Calories
	42.5 g protein
	9.5 g fat
	2.9 g fiber
	251 mg sodium
	46 g carbohydrate
UHEP	1/4 Vegetables & Fruit
	2 Grains
	1 Meat
	1/2 Milk

Ginger Chicken Stir-Fry

Stir-fry is one of the quickest dinners that I make. This recipe is great because while the chicken is marinating you are chopping up the veggies and cooking the rice! Multitasking in the kitchen, or what most of us call being "superwoman" or to be politically correct, "superperson."

2 cups / 500 mL **water**
1/2 cup / 125 mL **brown rice**
14 oz / 400 g **skinless boneless chicken breasts—cut on the diagonal into 1-in/2.5-cm slices**

Marinade
2 tbsp / 25 mL **light soy sauce**
2 tbsp / 25 mL **rice vinegar**
1 tbsp / 15 mL **honey**
1 tbsp / 15 mL **minced ginger**

Sauce
1 cup / 250 mL **vegetable stock or lower-sodium chicken stock**
2 **cloves garlic—minced**
2 tbsp / 25 mL **light soy sauce**
2 tbsp / 25 mL **honey**
1 tbsp / 15 mL **minced ginger**
1 tbsp / 15 mL **cornstarch**
1 tsp / 5 mL **chili garlic sauce** (see page 174)

Stir-Fry
2 **carrots—chopped on the diagonal into 1/2-in/1.2-cm slices**
2 cups / 500 mL **broccoli—chopped into florets**
2 cups / 500 mL **Chinese (Napa) cabbage—shredded**
1 cup / 250 mL **snow peas**
2 **green onions—chopped into 3-in/7.5-cm pieces**
1 **large red pepper—cut into 1-in/2.5-cm slices**
1 cup / 250 mL **bean sprouts—rinsed**
2 tsp / 10 mL **canola oil**

1   Boil the water and put in the rice. Return to boil. Cover and reduce to simmer. This will take 45 minutes.

2   Mix together the marinade ingredients. Add the sliced chicken. Cover with the marinade. Refrigerate for 15 to 20 minutes (or the time it takes you to chop up the veggies and cook the rice!)

3   Mix the sauce ingredients together. Set aside.

4   Prep the veggies.

5   Heat a large frying pan or wok. Add the canola oil. Remove the chicken from the marinade. Discard marinade. Stir-fry the chicken. When just cooked remove from the pan and reserve.

6   Stir-fry the carrots. Add the broccoli. Stir-fry till almost cooked.

7   Add the snow peas, red pepper and green onions. Continue to stir-fry.

8   Add the cooked chicken. Add the sauce to the pan. Stir till the sauce thickens. Add the bean sprouts. Toss. Serve over the rice.

Serves 4

ONE SERVING vegetable stock	385 Calories 37.1 g protein 7.0 g fat 6.3 g fiber 741 mg sodium 46 g carbohydrate
lower-sodium chicken stock	714 mg sodium
regular chicken stock	807 mg sodium
UHEP	1/2 Fat 3 1/2 Vegetables & Fruit 1 Grains 1 Meat

7/10 very sweet

Chicken with Dried Cranberries

The first time I ever tried a dried cranberry was at the Good Food Festival in Toronto back in 1999. They were a huge hit that year. The Festival is a weekend event that headlines new products to sample as well as cooking demonstrations to watch. All your favorite Canadian cooks are there, including yours truly! If you ever get to Toronto the first weekend in May, make sure to head down to the exhibits and eat your way through the show! In the meantime, pick up some dried cranberries at your grocery store!

14 oz / 400 g **skinless boneless chicken breasts—cut into 4 equal pieces**

Sauce
2 tbsp / 25 mL **orange marmalade**
2 tbsp / 25 mL **hot pepper jelly**
2 tbsp / 25 mL **frozen orange juice concentrate** (see page 165)
1 tbsp / 15 mL **balsamic vinegar**
1/2 cup / 125 mL **dried cranberries** (see page 257)

1   Preheat the oven to 450°F/230°C.

2   Line an 8 x 8-in/20 x 20-cm pan with parchment paper or foil. Lay the chicken on top.

3   In a medium bowl mix together the marmalade, hot pepper jelly, orange juice concentrate and balsamic vinegar.

4   Stir in the dried cranberries. Pour overtop the chicken.

5   Bake in the oven for 20 to 25 minutes or until the chicken is cooked.

6   When the chicken is cooked, pour off the liquid into a frying pan. Leave the chicken in the pan and cover. Bring the liquid to a boil and leave it to reduce for about 5 minutes until slightly thickened. Pour it over the chicken. Serve.

Serves 4

SERVING TIP
This goes great with regular brown rice or the Orange Bulgar recipe on page 183.

WHERE DO I FIND HOT PEPPER JELLY?
In the condiment aisle, along with some other terrific things like chutneys, curry pastes and ketchup!

ONE SERVING	283 Calories
	31.3 g protein
	3.7 g fat
	0.9 g fiber
	83 mg sodium
	30 g carbohydrate
UHEP	1/2 Vegetables & Fruit
	1 Meat

HOW DO I POACH A CHICKEN?

In the dead of night, sneak into the King's lands. Shoot a chicken, and run like . . . Okay—poaching chicken—here goes:

Bring 2 cups/500 mL chicken stock to a boil.

Add 4 skinless chicken breasts.

Cover the pan, reduce the heat to simmer, and gently simmer for 10 to 15 minutes or until just cooked.

Remove the chicken to cool. Save the stock. It will make all the recipes using stock taste that much better.

When the chicken is cool, remove the bones. Use as needed. Or buy a cooked chicken at the grocery store.

HOW DO I PEEL AND CHOP UP A MANGO?

Very carefully. Mango 101:

Hold the mango on its side.

With a sharp knife, slice lengthwise about 1/3 of the way in. You should just miss the pit. Do the same thing on the other side.

Make a cross-hatch pattern without cutting through the flesh.

Turn the fruit inside out.

It will look like a lot of rectangular shapes popping out! Cut these off close to the peel.

ONE SERVING	281 Calories
	18.5 g protein
	13.9 g fat
	4.3 g fiber
	70 mg sodium
	21 g carbohydrate
UHEP	1/2 Fat
	3 Vegetables & Fruit
	1/2 Meat
	1/2 Nuts

Chicken Mango Salad

My friend Michale told me about an amazing hot mustard chicken mango salad she had just eaten at a restaurant in LA. She described the flavors so well my mouth was watering. I thought about it all night, got up the next day and bought the ingredients. Here is my mouth-watering version of her restaurant experience.

3 oz / 85 g **cooked poached chicken—shredded**
1 **mango**
4 cups / 1 L **baby greens or mesclun mix**
1 **stalk celery—chopped**
1/4 cup / 50 mL **walnuts**

Dressing
1 tsp / 5 mL **extra virgin olive oil**
1 tsp / 5 mL **red wine vinegar**
2 tsp / 10 mL **horseradish mustard** (see page 213)
2 tbsp / 25 mL **low-fat yogurt**

1   Poach chicken—see sidebar. Shred using a fork.

2   Peel and chop the mango—see sidebar.

3   Whisk together all the dressing ingredients.

4   Divide the greens equally between two serving plates. Sprinkle with celery.

5   Divide the chicken, walnuts and mango equally between the two plates, pour on half of the dressing on each plate. Serve.

Serves 2

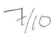
7/10

Grilled Chicken

Here are my two all-time favorite grilled chicken recipes. I use a resealable freezer-weight plastic bag to marinate the chicken in. No more juggling pans in the fridge or spilling the marinade all over the place. And there's nothing to clean up! You just throw out the bag! I love that part. I can't wait for someone to invent throwaway pots!

Lemon Chicken
Kid-Approved

14 oz / 400 g skinless boneless chicken breasts—cut into 4 equal pieces

Marinade
1 cup / 250 mL lemonade
4 cloves garlic—crushed
1 lemon—zest and juice of
freshly ground pepper
1 large resealable plastic bag

1   Four to 12 hours before cooking time—mix the lemonade, crushed garlic, zest and juice from 1 lemon, and the freshly ground pepper in the large resealable bag. Basically you are swishing all the ingredients in the bag!

2   Add the chicken. Here comes the crucial part—make sure the bag is really sealed! Give it a shake. Refrigerate for 4 to 12 hours.

3   Cooking time—heat up the grill or the barbecue.

4   Remove the chicken from the bag. Pour the liquid into a saucepan.

5   Grill the chicken slowly until no longer pink on the inside. Remember to use tongs to flip it.

6   While the chicken is grilling, heat the marinade in the saucepan. Bring to the boil. This is really important. You have to boil this gently for 15 minutes. Add more lemonade if it looks like you just may boil it all away!

7   Spoon this cooked marinade over the grilled chicken.

Serves 4

TIP
These two recipes are great to pack for the cottage or a camping trip. Put all the ingredients into the plastic bag, stick it in your cooler, fight the traffic to the cottage or campground, arrive 4 to 8 hours after leaving your home, get the barbecue going, have someone else cook the chicken while you make a salad, open a bottle of white wine, preferably a cold bottle of oaky Chardonnay, and enjoy your dinner. My idea of roughing it!

ONE SERVING	198 Calories
	31.3 g protein
	3.6 g fat
	0.3 g fiber
	76 mg sodium
	9 g carbohydrate
UHEP	1 Meat

WHERE DO I FIND 240 ML OF RASPBERRY COCKTAIL?
You find it in the juice aisle. It comes in a tetra pak sleeve of three. Great to have on hand— use one and save the other two for the next time you make this recipe, and believe me, you'll make it again and again.

KID TALK
Your kids don't like rosemary? Be a good parent and pick it off!

Raspberry Chicken
Kid-Approved

I have always wondered why the person who stands at the barbecue turning the food takes all the credit for how wonderful the food tastes. Now, I do agree that without turning the food on a regular basis, you would have burnt offerings, but any "cook" knows that most of the flavor comes from the marinade. So if your barbecuer starts taking the credit for this wonderful chicken, tell them Mairlyn should be taking the credit!

14 oz / 400 g **skinless boneless chicken breasts—cut into 4 equal pieces**

Marinade
1 240 mL **raspberry cocktail**
1/4 cup / 50 mL **raspberry vinegar**
2 tbsp / 25 mL **fresh rosemary**
1 **large resealable plastic bag**

1 Combine the raspberry cocktail, raspberry vinegar and fresh rosemary in a resealable plastic bag.

2 Add the chicken. Seal the bag and shake. Refrigerate for 8 to 12 hours.

3 Heat barbecue or grill.

4 Remove chicken from the marinade. Reserve liquid.

5 Grill chicken over medium-low heat until cooked.

6 Meanwhile, pour the marinade into a saucepan. Throw out the bag.

7 Bring the marinade to the boil and then reduce to simmer. Simmer for 15 minutes or until thick. It's important to simmer for 15 minutes to ensure that the marinade is thoroughly cooked.)

8 Pour cooked marinade over cooked chicken and serve.

Serves 4

ONE SERVING	197 Calories
	31.1 g protein
	3.6 g fat
	0.1 g fiber
	75 mg sodium
	9 g carbohydrate
UHEP	1 Meat

8/10 - didn't stay together

Chicken Burgers

Kid-Approved

The first time I had a chicken burger, I thought, you've got to be kidding. It was tasteless, fell apart and had a less than wonderful texture. I immediately rushed home and began working on a chicken burger that was edible. Okay, maybe it was a day later, but the point is, I had to make one that was better. It's a weird thing some of us do. Like tasting food in restaurants and trying to figure out what's in it! I really ought to get a life!

2 slices **whole-wheat bread**
1/4 cup / 50 mL **ketchup**
2 tbsp / 25 mL **vinegar**
1 tbsp / 15 mL **brown sugar**
1/4 tsp / 1 mL **cayenne**
1 **onion—minced**
1 **egg**
1 lb / 450 g **lean ground chicken**

1 Preheat barbecue.

2 Using a blender or food processor make the whole-wheat bread into crumbs.

3 In a large bowl mix the rest of the ingredients with the crumbs. Shape into 6 burgers.

4 Grill on barbecue until cooked through.

5 Serve on a whole-wheat hamburger bun with the burger fixings, mustard, relish, ketchup and low-fat mayo, or eat as a bunless burger! Not as much fun, but a big calorie-saver.

Serves 6

ONE SERVING on a hamburger bun	271 Calories
	22.1 g protein
	10.4 g fat
	3.0 g fiber
	378 mg sodium
	30 g carbohydrate
UHEP	2 1/4 Grains
	1 Meat

ONE SERVING not on a hamburger bun	158 Calories
	17.9 g protein
	7.8 g fat
	1.3 g fiber
	182 mg sodium
	11 g carbohydrate
UHEP	1/4 Grains
	1 Meat

Salsa Baked Chicken

I have been a huge fan of salsa since I first discovered it while I was going to acting school in Pasadena, California. Once I tried it, I was hooked. I put it on everything, including my scrambled eggs, which I still do. I once had a chicken dish at a restaurant down there and have been making my version of it ever since.

1 1/4 cups / 300 mL **commercial salsa—medium to hot**
1/2 cup / 125 mL **Dijon mustard**
1 **lime—juice and zest of**
4 **cloves garlic—minced**
14 oz / 400 g **skinless boneless chicken breasts—cut into 4 equal pieces**

1 Preheat the oven to 425°F/220°C.

2 In a bowl mix together the salsa, Dijon mustard, lime juice, zest and garlic.

3 Line a 8 x 8-in/20 x 20-cm pan with parchment paper. (Do not use tin foil—it will make this dish taste metallic. Use parchment paper.) Place chicken breasts in pan. Cover with the salsa mixture.

4 Bake for 20 to 25 minutes or until done, basting once or twice.

5 Serve. Pour the sauce over the chicken and serve with brown rice or bulgar.

Serves 4

ONE SERVING	227 Calories
	32.5 g protein
	3.6 g fat
	0.3 g fiber
	74 mg sodium
	10 g carbohydrate
UHEP	1/2 Vegetables & Fruit
	1 Meat

Seafood

7/10

Wasabi Salmon

WHAT IS WASABI AND WHERE CAN I BUY IT?

Wasabi is a green horseradish that is used in Japanese cooking, especially in sushi. It has a very hot effect, very different from regular spicy food. Wasabi goes right up to the top of your head, and can make you feel as if your head just blew off your shoulders! It is very distinctive, and once you've tried it, you are either hooked, or not. I'm one of the hooked ones!

WHY SHORT-GRAIN BROWN RICE?

Short grain gives you a stickier rice than long grain and is more like traditional sticky Japanese rice.

Okay, I'll admit it, I'm really bossy. When my friend Michale and I cook I am always telling her what to do, and she is usually telling me off!

I had always thought that a wasabi salmon dish would be terrific. I could almost taste the flavors in my mind. The first time I made it, surprisingly enough, it wasn't even hot. Michale thought that reserving some of the wasabi sauce to drizzle over the fish would do the trick and for once I went along with her. And you know, she was right! Reserve some for the final drizzle.

13 oz / 370 g **salmon fillet**
2 tsp / 10 mL **wasabi paste or powder**
2 tsp / 10 mL **light soy sauce**
2 tsp / 10 mL **rice vinegar**
2 tsp / 10 mL **minced fresh ginger**
1 tbsp / 15 mL **dark brown sugar**

1. Preheat oven to 425°F/220°C.
2. Line a 8 x 8-in/20 x 20-cm pan with parchment paper or foil.
3. Place salmon in the pan.
4. In a small bowl mix together the wasabi paste, soy sauce, rice vinegar, fresh ginger and brown sugar. Reserve 2 tsp/10 mL.
5. Pour remaining sauce overtop of the fish. Bake in the oven for 15 to 20 minutes or until just done.
6. When cooked, pour the reserved wasabi sauce over the fish and serve with short-grain brown rice.

Serves 4

ONE SERVING without rice	186 Calories 18.6 g protein 10.0 g fat 0.1 g fiber 196 mg sodium 4 g carbohydrate
UHEP	1 Fish

Spicy Salmon Cakes

My best friend Michale and her husband have a cottage in Muskoka. Most weekends in the summer you can find us discussing the ins and outs of child rearing, the annoying habits of our loved ones, how perfect we are and what we're going to eat next, not nesessarily in that order.

I had been working on this salmon cake recipe for a while and it was ready for an official taste test. I was making eight dishes that night so Michale suggested we make the salmon cakes appetizer-size and serve them with dipping sauces. They were most excellent and here are the recipes! I still like them best as a main course, but they are also great as an appetizer.

28 **Triscuits—50% less salt—reserve** 1/2 cup / 125 mL **for coating**
2 7.5-oz / 213-g **cans salmon—well drained**
2 tbsp / 25 mL **low-fat mayonnaise**
2 tbsp / 25 mL **low-fat plain yogurt**
1 tbsp / 15 mL **Dijon mustard**
1/2 tsp / 2 mL **Worcestershire sauce**
2 tsp / 10 mL **chili garlic sauce** (see page 174)
1/2 **sweet onion—minced**
1/2 **red pepper—minced**
1/4 cup / 50 mL **finely chopped cilantro**
1 tbsp / 15 mL **fresh lime juice**

1   Preheat the oven to 425°F/220°C.

2   In a food processor, crush up the Triscuits. Set aside 1/2 cup/125 mL to use as the coating.

3   Put the salmon in the food processor and pulse several times.

4   Add the mayonnaise, yogurt, Worcestershire sauce, chili garlic sauce, onion and red pepper. Pulse until well combined.

5   Add the cilantro and the lime juice and pulse till combined.

6   Form into 14 salmon cakes. Roll in the reserved crumbs. Place on a cookie sheet lined with parchment paper.

7   Bake for 10 minutes. Flip over and bake for 10 more minutes. Serve with or without Michale's Dipping Sauces (next page).

Serves 7

NO FOOD PROCESSOR?
Crush the Triscuits with a rolling pin and mix all the other ingredients together in a large bowl. Put a food processor on your wish list.

ONE SERVING	214 Calories
2 cakes without sauce	13.0 g protein
	10.6 g fat
	2.4 g fiber
	426 mg sodium
	16 g carbohydrate
UHEP	3/4 Fat
	1 Fish
	1 Grains

Michale's Dipping Sauces for Salmon Cakes

WHAT THE HECK IS HORSERADISH MUSTARD AND WHERE DO I FIND IT?
It is a Dijon mustard mixed with horseradish which gives it a real kick. You can find it with all the other mustards in most grocery stores.

Michale's Dippy Sauce

3 tbsp / 45 mL **low-fat mayonnaise**
1 tbsp / 15 mL **horseradish mustard**
1 tbsp / 15 mL **lemon juice**

1 Mix together in a small bowl. Serve.

Citrus Dipping Sauce

3 tbsp / 45 mL **ketchup**
1 tbsp / 15 mL **orange juice concentrate**
1/4 tsp / 1 mL **Worcestershire sauce**

1 Mix together in a small bowl. Serve.

ONE SERVING	237 Calories
2 cakes with Dippy Sauce	13.0 g protein
	12.8 g fat
	2.4 g fiber
	426 mg sodium
	17 g carbohydrate
UHEP	2 Fat
	1 Fish
	1 Grains
ONE SERVING	226 Calories
2 cakes with Citrus Sauce	13.2 g protein
	10.6 g fat
	2.5 g fiber
	474 mg sodium
	19 g carbohydrate
UHEP	3/4 Fat
	1 Fish
	1 Grains

Baked Salmon with Fresh Citrus

How simple can a recipe get? Five ingredients and a salmon fillet? And it's ready in 30 minutes or less? Welcome to a simple supper that can pass off as elegant anytime. This is a family favorite that I also serve to company. It always gets raves! And—that is one of the main reasons that we cook, isn't it?

1 **lime**
1 **lemon**
1 **orange**
3 tbsp / 45 mL **honey**
1 tbsp / 15 mL **finely grated fresh ginger**
13 oz / 370 g **salmon fillet**

1   Preheat oven to 425°F/220°C.

2   Line an 8 x 8-in/20 x 20-cm pan with parchment paper or foil.

3   Zest the lime, lemon and orange. Set zest aside.

4   Juice the lime, lemon and orange. Mix the juices together. Add the honey and ginger.

5   Lay the salmon in the pan. Pour the citrus/honey/ginger mixture overtop. Sprinkle with the zests. See sidebar.

6   Bake for 15 to 20 minutes or until just done. Remove salmon from the pan and cover. Pour off the sauce into a pan. Bring to a boil and reduce by half.

7   Serve with brown rice. Spoon the sauce over the salmon and rice.

Serves 4

HOW DO I KNOW WHETHER OR NOT THE FISH IS FRESH?

Well, first of all, if it's smelly don't buy it! Remember the rule of thumb—fresh fish should smell like the ocean. Clean and fresh. Not like low tide. Smelly and stale. Another rule when buying fresh fish—look to see that the flesh is firm to the touch. Ask the fishmonger to poke the fish. Ask nicely! The pressure of a finger shouldn't leave an impression in the flesh! If it does, say you forgot your keys in the car and walk away. When buying a whole fish—check to see that the eyes are bulging out and clear. If sunken and cloudy, go with the lost keys story.

SO WHAT DOES "UNTIL JUST DONE" MEAN ANYWAY?

Well, when it comes to fish, it means when the fish just starts to flake or separate when you prod it with a fork. Overcooked fish falls apart easily and is very dry. "Until just done" fish is tender, juicy, and melts in your mouth!

KID-FRIENDLY TIP

"What's That Funny Looking Stuff on Top of the Fish?" If you think that your child is going to be zest-challenged, leave it off, or scrape it off just before serving.

WHY 13 OZ NOT 12 OZ?

Shrinkage!

ONE SERVING without rice	218 Calories
	18.7 g protein
	10.1 g fat
	0.5 g fiber
	56 mg sodium
	18 g carbohydrate
UHEP	1 Fish
	1/4 Vegetables & Fruit

Company's Comin' Salmon

TIP

If the foil won't keep its shape around the fish, lightly crinkle up a large piece of foil and place it between the foil pouch and the side of the pan.

As I have mentioned before, the trick to really good salmon is really fresh salmon. It should smell clean like the ocean, without any hint of a "fishy" odor. If you walk into a fish store that makes you want to faint from the odors, leave!

13 oz / 370 g **salmon fillet**

Poaching Liquid
1/2 cup / 125 mL **dry white wine**
1/4 cup / 50 mL **orange juice concentrate** (see page 165)
1/2 tbsp / 7.5 mL **lime juice**
1 **shallot—diced**
1 tsp / 5 mL **mixed peppercorns**

1 Preheat oven to 425°F/220°C.

2 Line a 8 x 8-in/20 x 20-cm pan with parchment paper or foil.

3 Cut the salmon fillet into 4 equal pieces, place in the pan.

4 In a small bowl mix together the white wine, orange juice concentrate, lime juice, shallot and peppercorns.

5 Place the fillets in the pan, leaving 1/2 in/1 cm between the pieces.

6 Pour the poaching liquid overtop. Pull up the sides of the foil to make sure the poaching liquid stays close to the salmon.

7 Bake in the oven for 15 to 20 minutes or until just done.

Serves 4

ONE SERVING	182 Calories
	18.5 g protein
	10.0 g fat
	0 g fiber
	55 mg sodium
	2 g carbohydrate
UHEP	1 Fish

9/10!

Baked Salmon with Fresh Ginger

I was born and raised in Vancouver, on salmon! An old fishmonger drove around the neighborhood on Fridays in a beat-up truck selling salmon, shrimp, cod, sole and sometimes crab. The bed of the truck had a flat metal top with three holes in it that were covered while he drove around ringing his bell. When you stopped him, he would open up the covered holes to reveal freshly caught fish packed in ice. You would pick out the one that you wanted, he would expertly cut off how much you wanted, weigh it, wrap it in brown paper and then tell you how much you owed him. The "fish man" as my mother called him was very old and rather scary-looking to me, but boy oh boy did he have fresh fish!

13 oz / 370 g **salmon fillet**
1/4 cup / 50 mL **Dijon mustard**
1/4 cup / 50 mL **dark brown sugar**
3 tbsp / 45 mL **light soy sauce**
3 tbsp / 45 mL **rice vinegar**
1 tbsp / 15 mL **grated fresh ginger**
1 **medium onion—finely minced**
1/4 tsp / 1 mL **red pepper flakes**

1   Preheat oven to 425°F/220°C.

2   Line a 8 x 8-in/20 x 20-cm pan with parchment paper or foil.

3   Place salmon in the pan.

4   In a medium bowl mix together the Dijon mustard, brown sugar, soy sauce, rice vinegar, grated ginger, minced onion and red pepper flakes. Pour overtop of the salmon.

5   Bake in the oven for 15 to 20 minutes or until just done. Baste.

6   Serve with brown rice. Spoon the sauce over the rice and the fish.

Serves 4

ONE SERVING without rice	255 Calories
	19.6 g protein
	10.1 g fat
	0.4 g fiber
	691 mg sodium
	19 g carbohydrate
UHEP	1 Fish

Salmon with Mango Salsa

KID-FRIENDLY TIP
Omit the salsa. Serve the fish
with some slices of mango and
red pepper on the side.

The salsa in this recipe is amazing. The colors of the red pepper and the mango remind me of summer.

Salsa
1 **large ripe mango—diced** (see page 205)
1/2 **red pepper—diced**
1 **lime—juice of**
2 tbsp / 25 mL **finely chopped chives**
1/4 tsp / 1 mL **red pepper flakes**
13 oz / 370 g **salmon fillet**

1 In a bowl mix together the diced mango, red pepper, lime juice, chives and red pepper flakes.

2 Cover and set aside for up to 1 day in advance. If you are making this the day ahead, refrigerate it. If not it's okay to leave it on the counter, covered, for up to 30 minutes.

3 Heat your indoor or outdoor grill.

4 Cut the fillet into 4 equal pieces.

5 Cook the salmon on the grill until just cooked. Avoid cooking the living daylights out of it. Most people don't like fish because they had a bad overcooked fillet experience. Cook it just until the meat starts to flake easily. This should take about 5 to 10 minutes per side depending on how thick the fillet is.

6 Serve with the mango/salsa mixture on the top of each fillet.

Serves 4

ONE SERVING	201 Calories
	18.5 g protein
	10.0 g fat
	0.7 g fiber
	56 mg sodium
	8 g carbohydrate
UHEP	1 Fish
	1/2 Vegetables & Fruit

Poached Salmon with Mairlyn's World Famous Lime Mayo

Kid-Approved

I have been making this poached salmon for about 20 years. I guess that means I can't tell people that I'm 34 anymore. No...I started cooking at 14, yeah, that's the ticket—14!

Anyway, it is a cinch to make, always gets raves, and you can make it any time of the year. In the summertime poach it and then chill it and it becomes—cold poached salmon! So hot or cold, it's a winner. Always serve with my World Famous Lime Mayo.

2 cups / 500 mL **orange juice**
13 oz / 370 g **salmon fillet—cut into 4 equal pieces**

World Famous Lime Mayo
2 tbsp + 2 tsp / 35 mL **low-fat mayonnaise**
1 **lime—juice of**

1 In a covered frying pan, bring the orange juice to a boil.

2 When the juice begins to boil, add the salmon. The juice should just cover the fillets. Cover with the lid.

3 Reduce heat and gently poach for 5 to 10 minutes.

4 Meanwhile, mix together the mayonnaise and the lime juice. Set aside.

5 Check to see if the salmon is cooked through.

6 When cooked, remove salmon using a slotted spoon. Serve with the sauce overtop.

Serves 4

SERVING COLD

If serving as a cold poached salmon, poach it whole, preferably wrapped loosely in cheesecloth. Carefully lift the cooked salmon out of the poaching liquid onto a plate. Let cool. Remove cheesecloth. Cover in plastic wrap and store in the fridge for up to 24 hours. At serving time drizzle with my World Famous Lime Mayo and garnish with slices of lime.

WORLD FAMOUS LIME MAYO

I did a fair amount of catering back in the '70s and '80s, mostly for family and friends. I would have tons of gorgeous foods out and always a salmon with my World Famous Lime Mayo. Afterwards, someone would always ask me for the recipe for the sauce. I never gave it away, not because it was such a big secret, but because I didn't want anyone to know how simple it was!

ONE SERVING	204 Calories
	18.4 g protein
	13.3 g fat
	0 g fiber
	54 mg sodium
	1 g carbohydrate
UHEP	1/2 Fat
	1 Fish

Salmon Teriyaki

KID-FRIENDLY TIP

Most kids won't eat the ginger that is on top of the fish. Either scrape it off when you serve it or make sure that it isn't on top of the fish before you bake it, which is tricky. But all parents figure this kind of thing out eventually!

My West Coast specialty. I've always maintained that most fish abstainers have just never eaten really fantastic fish! Case in point—I served this on a Canada Day long weekend up at Michale's cottage last summer and Susan, a long-suffering salmon slagger, had seconds! I love when that happens.

13 oz / 370 g **salmon fillet**
2 tbsp / 25 mL **sodium-reduced soy sauce**
2 tbsp / 25 mL **rice vinegar**
2 tbsp / 25 mL **brown sugar**
2 tsp / 10 mL **grated fresh ginger**

1   Preheat oven to 425°F/220°C.

2   Line an 8 x 8-in/20 x 20-cm pan with parchment paper or foil.

3   Place salmon in the pan.

4   Mix together the soy sauce, rice vinegar, brown sugar and fresh ginger. Pour over the fish.

5   Bake for 15 to 20 minutes or until fish is just done. Serve with brown rice and spoon the sauce overtop.

Serves 4

ONE SERVING	191 Calories
without rice	18.9 g protein
	10.0 g fat
	0 g fiber
	476 mg sodium
	5 g carbohydrate
UHEP	1 Fish

"Really Great Salmon!"

Every time I serve this, people say, "Hey, this is really great salmon!" So, I thought, what the heck—it may not be the most creative name for a recipe, but it really is "really great salmon!"

13 oz / 370 g **salmon fillet**
2 tbsp / 25 mL **sodium-reduced soy sauce**
1 tsp / 5 mL **Worcestershire sauce**
1/4 tsp / 1 mL **dry mustard**
1/4 tsp / 2 mL **pepper**
1 **clove garlic—minced**

per person

1   Preheat oven to 425°F/220°C.

2   Line an 8 x 8-in/20 x 20-cm pan with parchment paper or foil.

3   Place salmon in the pan.

4   Mix together the soy sauce, Worcestershire sauce, dry mustard, pepper and minced garlic. Pour over the salmon fillet.

5   Bake for 15 to 20 minutes or until just done. Spoon the sauce over the salmon and serve with brown rice.

Serves 4

KID-FRIENDLY TIP
FILLET OR STEAK?
I always buy fillets. I find that without the hassle of "bone excavation" my son will eat a fillet in a minute. Even though they are more money, you only need 3 oz/85 g for 1 serving, and a fillet gets all eaten. A steak, on the other hand, has a fair amount of waste, then there is the need to check for bones and the whole "skin thing." Andrew, my son, won't even have the skin on his plate, and he's not a picky eater! So, when I weigh out the pros and cons, I always end up buying the fillets.

ONE SERVING *without rice*	180 Calories
	19.0 g protein
	10.0 g fat
	0.1 g fiber
	486 mg sodium
	2 g carbohydrate
UHEP	1 Fish

Creamy Dilled Salmon

KID-FRIENDLY TIP

Leaving the dill out of the recipe is a bad idea, but let's face it, a lot of kids won't eat the "green stuff" on top of the salmon. Once again, my suggestion is to scrape it off at serving time. What we do for our kids! Hope they thank us for their good health when they are all grown up!

SERVING TIP

Spoon any extra sauce over whole-wheat pasta.

Oven-roasting fish is truly the fast food of the century. Most fish recipes can be prepared and served within 30 minutes. Now that's "fast food!"

13 oz / 370 g **salmon fillet**
1/4 cup / 50 mL **buttermilk**
3 tbsp / 45 mL **chopped fresh dill**
1 tbsp / 15 mL **Dijon mustard**
1 tbsp / 15 mL **orange juice concentrate** (see page 165)

1 Preheat oven to 425°F/220°C.

2 Line an 8 x 8-in/20 x 20-cm pan with parchment paper or foil.

3 Place salmon in the pan.

4 Mix together the buttermilk, chopped dill, Dijon mustard and orange juice concentrate. Pour over the salmon.

5 Bake for 15 to 20 minutes or until just done.

Serves 4

ONE SERVING *without pasta*	186 Calories
	19.0 g protein
	10.2 g fat
	0.1 g fiber
	70 mg sodium
	3 g carbohydrate
UHEP	1 Fish

6/10 - Kind of borring.

Sunset Shrimp

As I've mentioned before, I tested many recipes at my friend's cottage. On one of the many testing nights— wine, 14 people and mosquitoes, I came up with this shrimp dish. Our friend, David, was looking at the sunset at the time and said that the flavors made him feel like the sunset. It's surprising what you can say when drinking red wine. Anyway, I thought he was fairly whacked, so I tried it, and darned if he was right. This fiery shrimp dish does taste like a Muskoka Sunset, if and only if, you are drinking red wine!

1 1/2 cups / 375 mL **whole-wheat spaghetti**
1 tbsp / 15 mL **extra virgin olive oil**
40 **medium shrimp—cleaned**
1/3 cup / 75 mL **Chardonnay**
1 tsp / 5 mL **chili garlic sauce** (see page 174)
1/2 **red pepper—minced**
1 **green onion—diced**
1/3 cup / 75 mL **cilantro—finely chopped**

1   Put water on to boil in a large pot. When boiling, add the whole-wheat spaghetti and cook for 9 to 10 minutes or until tender.

2   In a nonstick frying pan heat the oil. Add the shrimp and cook quickly. Remove after the shrimps have turned pink. Set aside.

3   Add the Chardonnay, chili garlic sauce and red pepper. Stir and let the red pepper cook for 1 minute.

4   Add the cooked shrimp, green onion and cilantro. Stir. Remove from heat.

5   Drain the cooked pasta. Divide equally among four plates.

6   Divide the shrimp equally. Pour the sauce over and serve.

Serves 4

ONE SERVING	300 Calories
	23.0 g protein
	6.0 g fat
	3.0 g fiber
	147 mg sodium
	34 g carbohydrate
UHEP	3/4 Fat
	1 1/2 Grains
	1 Fish

Salmon Chowder

Kid-Approved

QUICK TIP

Next time salmon is on sale, buy an extra 13 oz/370 g, cube it into 1-in/2.5-cm pieces and freeze in a freezer bag. Making the chowder for dinner? Take out the frozen cubes, drop the bag and all into a sink full of cold water, and it will be thawed out in about 20 minutes. Or defrost them in the bag in your microwave.

A complete meal in a bowl! Add a 100% whole-wheat bun and you have all the food groups present and accounted for. And it's ready in 30 minutes! Who says eating well has to be difficult?

3 cups / 750 mL **chicken stock or lower-sodium chicken stock**
1 **medium onion—diced**
3 **cloves garlic—minced**
3 **large carrots—chopped**
2 **stalks celery—chopped**
1 **red pepper—chopped**
1 **small potato—diced**
1 cup / 250 mL **corn kernels—fresh or frozen**
13 oz / 370 g **salmon fillet—skinned**
1 cup / 250 mL **fat-free evaporated milk**

1 Put chicken stock, onion, garlic and carrots into a large pot. Bring to the boil.

2 Add the celery, red pepper, potatoes and corn. Stir in well.

3 Bring back to the boil. Reduce the heat to simmer. Cover and simmer for 10 minutes. The veggies should be cooked.

4 Cube the salmon into 1-in/2.5-cm cubes. Add to the pot and simmer, covered, for 5 minutes or until the salmon is just cooked.

5 Add the fat-free evaporated milk. Stir till combined. Add pepper to taste. Serve.

Serves 4

ONE SERVING	333 Calories
	28.0 g protein
	10.4 g fat
	4.5 g fiber
	890 mg sodium
	33 g carbohydrate
lower-sodium chicken stock	611 mg sodium
UHEP	1 Fish
	3 1/4 Vegetables & Fruit
	1/2 Milk

Beef

Beef and Broccoli Stir-Fry

Kid-Approved

This first time I tried out this recipe was when my son's friend, Robert, was at our house for a sleepover, an eleven-year-old's idea of a great night, and a mother's nightmare! Before they ended up playing tackle football in Andrew's room at 11:23 p.m., they both wolfed down this stir-fry. Serves 4, and two eleven-year-olds ate the whole thing.

Marinade

2 tbsp / 25 mL **sodium-reduced soy sauce**
2 tbsp / 25 mL **oyster sauce**
2 tbsp / 25 mL **rice vinegar**
2 tbsp / 25 mL **water**
14 oz / 400 g **top sirloin steak—sliced thinly**

Sauce

1 cup / 250 mL **beef stock**
6 tbsp / 90 mL **oyster sauce**
1/4 cup / 50 mL **rice vinegar**
1 tsp / 5 mL **chili garlic sauce** (see page 174)
1/2 tsp / 2 mL **sugar**
1 tbsp + 1 tsp / 20 mL **cornstarch**

1 tbsp + 1 tsp / 20 mL **extra virgin olive oil**
2 **onions—sliced thinly**
4 cups / 1 L **broccoli florets**
4 **cloves garlic**

1 Mix together the marinade ingredients. Add the thinly sliced beef. Marinate for 30 minutes.

2 Mix together the sauce ingredients and set aside.

3 When the meat has marinated, drain, heat a large non-stick frying pan or a wok. When hot add the beef and stir-fry till just done. Remove from pan and set aside. Discard any liquid.

4 Reheat the pan and add the olive oil. Stir-fry the onions and broccoli for 3 minutes. Add the garlic and beef. Stir till heated through.

5 Restir the sauce ingredients and add to pan, stirring until thick.

6 Serve over brown rice.

Serves 4

ONE SERVING	275 Calories
without rice	33.8 g protein
	10.7 g fat
	3.4 g fiber
	455 mg sodium
	12 g carbohydrate
UHEP	1 Fat
	2 Vegetables & Fruit
	1 Meat

Beef Kebobs

Kid-Approved

The only difficult part to this recipe is making sure that you seal the resealable bag so it doesn't explode on you when you squish it. It can happen. I speak from experience. Make extra sure the resealable bag really is sealed.

Marinade

1 9-oz / 250-mL carton **V8 cocktail**
1/3 cup / 75 mL **red wine vinegar**
3 tbsp / 45 mL **brown sugar**
2 tbsp / 25 mL **ketchup**
1 tbsp / 15 mL **extra virgin olive oil**
1 tbsp / 15 mL **Worcestershire sauce**
1 tsp / 5 mL **chili powder**
1/4 tsp / 1 mL **cayenne** — *too much!*
4 **cloves garlic—crushed**
14 oz / 400 g **top sirloin steak—cut into 12 equal pieces**

2 **red peppers—cut into 8 pieces**
2 **orange peppers—cut into 8 pieces**
8 **mushrooms**
2 **red onions—cut into 8 pieces**
4 **large metal skewers**

A 9-OZ (250-ML) CARTON OF V8?

For all you people who don't want to buy the 1 L of V8—go to the juice aisle and buy the 3 x 250 mL tetra pak cartons of it. You only use one per recipe and the rest can be stored in your pantry till the next time you want to kebob.

1 Mix all the marinade ingredients in a large resealable plastic bag. Reserve 1/4 cup/50 mL.

2 Put the steak into the bag.

3 Seal the bag and shake it to make sure that the meat is coated with liquid.

4 Put the bag in the refrigerator for 8 hours or up to 24 hours.

5 At cooking time—heat barbecue to medium.

6 Remove the meat from the bag, discarding marinade.

7 Assemble kebobs—be creative. Use 3 pieces of meat, 2 pieces of red pepper, 2 pieces of orange pepper, 2 mushrooms and 2 pieces of onion per skewer.

8 Put on the barbecue, baste with reserved marinade and grill till meat is cooked—about 5 minutes.

9 Serve with a green salad and brown rice.

Serves 4

ONE SERVING kebob only	273 Calories 33.4 g protein 6.9 g fat 3.7 g fiber 96 mg sodium 20 g carbohydrate
UHEP	2 1/2 Vegetables & Fruit 1 Meat

Beans

Summer Fiesta Chickpea Salad

I've made many bean salads in my day—boy does that sound like a line or what? Well, it's the truth, I have made a lot of different bean salads and this one is my favorite. It's colorful and the dressing is light and fresh-tasting. Lasts for up to 3 days in the fridge.

1 19-oz / 540-mL can **chickpeas—drained and rinsed**
1 **large red pepper—diced**
1 **large orange pepper—diced**
2 cups / 500 mL **grape tomatoes—cut into halves**
3 **green onions—chopped finely**
1 **stalk celery—sliced thinly**
3 **cloves garlic—minced**

Dressing
1 tbsp + 1 tsp / 20 mL **extra virgin olive oil**
1 tbsp + 1 tsp / 20 mL **red wine vinegar**
1 tbsp / 15 mL **Dijon mustard**
1 tsp / 5 mL **honey**

1   In a large bowl mix together the chickpeas, red pepper, orange pepper, grape tomatoes, green onions, celery and minced garlic.

2   In a separate bowl mix together the olive oil, red wine vinegar, Dijon mustard and honey.

3   Pour the dressing over the salad and mix till well-combined. Cover and refrigerate for 30 minutes or up to 1 week.

4   Serve over chopped romaine lettuce.

Serves 4

ONE SERVING	258 Calories
	8.5 g protein
	6.7 g fat
	8.5 g fiber
	221 mg sodium
	43 g carbohydrate
UHEP	1 Beans
	1 Fat
	2 3/4 Vegetables & Fruit

Hummus with Roasted Red Peppers

WHAT THE HECK IS TAHINI AND WHERE DO I FIND IT?

Tahini is sesame seed paste. You can find it in the international foods section in your grocery store or at any health food store. Once you open the bottle store it in the fridge for up to 6 months. Once you've tried this recipe, it won't be kicking around the back of your fridge that long.

HOW DO I EAT HUMMUS?

I put hummus into a whole-wheat pita and then stuff it with sprouts, chopped tomato and lettuce. Liz likes to make sandwiches out of hers using whole-wheat bread. As another idea—we both serve it as a dip with raw veggies.

This recipe took me forever to create. I know, I know, hummus is easy to make, how could it have taken forever? Well for starters, I tried making it without tahini. Big mistake. Hummus without tahini is like the Beatles without John.

I also tried adding way too much other stuff. At one point I was trying to convince my assistant, Dawn, the Hummus Queen, that adding parsley and sesame oil was a really good idea. She took one taste and said, very quietly, "I can't really taste the chickpeas." She was right. I couldn't taste them either.

I labored away, and finally came up with this very simple version of hummus that tastes, according to Dawn, "really, really great."

1 19 oz / 540 mL can **chickpeas—drained and rinsed**
2 tbsp / 25 mL **tahini**
2 tbsp / 25 mL **lemon juice**
1/8 tsp / 0.5 mL **cayenne**
2 **cloves garlic**
3 tbsp / 45 mL **water**
2 **whole roasted red peppers** (see page 193)

1 In a food processor or blender purée all the ingredients, except the red pepper, together. Purée till very smooth. Then add the red pepper and pulse till well combined.

2 Store covered in the fridge for up to 1 week.

Serves 8. Makes 2 cups/500 mL.

ONE SERVING	117 Calories
	4.5 g protein
	3.0 g fat
	3.8 g fiber
	102 mg sodium
	19 g carbohydrate
UHEP	1/2 Beans
	3/4 Fat
	1/2 Vegetables & Fruit

Mairlyn's World Famous Beans and Rice

I became a vegetarian while I was in second year at university in the '70s. I had this really cute young-looking prof who encouraged us to try vegetarianism. It turned out that this hunk of manhood was in fact in his late 60s. I figured I would do whatever it took to look as good as he did at that age and, being truly vain in my 20s, I became a vegetarian the next day.

This is one of my "famous" recipes! It is truly fantastic! I know some of you will be less than enthusastic to try the bean recipes, but you would be missing out on the best chapter in the book. The recipes are all tasty, easy to make and easy to eat.

Although I am no longer a vegetarian (I eat fish and poultry), I love my beans. We eat them at least 3 to 5 times a week. Try all the recipes in this chapter—they are all "World Famous!"

1 tbsp + 1 tsp / 20 mL **extra virgin olive oil**
1 **onion—diced**
4 **cloves garlic—minced**
1 cup / 250 mL **long-grain brown rice**
1 28 oz / 796 mL **can plum tomatoes**
2 19 oz / 540 mL **cans red kidney beans—drained and rinsed**
1 cup / 250 mL **vegetable stock or lower-sodium chicken stock**
1 **orange pepper—coarsely chopped**
2 tsp / 10 mL **cumin**
1 1/2 tsp / 7 mL **coriander**
1/2 tsp / 2 mL **red pepper flakes**
3 cups / 750 mL **chopped kale**

WHY DRAIN AND RINSE THE BEANS?

Canned beans are much more convenient than soaking and cooking the dried variety. The only drawback is that canned beans are fairly high in sodium. When you drain and rinse them well you eliminate at least half of the salt.

WHY DO BEANS GIVE ME GAS AND WHAT THE HECK IS BEANO?

Indigestible sugars in the beans give you gas. What you can't digest makes you toot! Experts agree that the best way to cut down on gas is to eat beans more frequently, so your digestive system gets used to them. Remember there is always Beano—a commercial enzyme that helps digest those gas-producing sugars. Buy it at the drugstore and follow the directions for flatulent-free evenings!

1 Heat a large pot. Add the oil and the onion. Sauté for 2 minutes.

2 Add the garlic and sauté, stirring often to prevent burning. (It can happen really fast and burnt garlic tastes awful!)

3 Add the brown rice. Stir till coated.

4 Add the can of tomatoes, kidney beans and stock. Remember you have already drained and rinsed the beans, because you read the recipe through before you started!

5 Add the orange pepper, cumin, coriander and red pepper flakes.

6 Bring to the boil. Cover and reduce the heat to low. Simmer for 45 minutes or until the rice is cooked.

7 Remove the kale leaves from the stalks. Discard stalks. Chop leaves, add to the pot and stir well. Cover and simmer for 15 minutes or until the rice is cooked.

8 Serve with a green salad.

9 Never serve this on a first date!

Serves 8

ONE SERVING	275 Calories
approx. 3/4 cup/175 mL	11.4 g protein
	4.1 g fat
	12.9 g fiber
vegetable stock	562 mg sodium
	49 g carbohydrate
lower-sodium chicken stock	548 mg sodium
regular chicken stock	595 mg sodium
UHEP	1 Beans
	1/2 Fat
	1 1/2 Vegetables & Fruit
	3/4 Grains

Remarkable Refried Beans

Most cans of refried beans are loaded with lard! A big
fat no-no. Mine have only 1 tsp/5 mL of extra virgin
olive oil, making them a healthier choice.

Use the beans as a dip with vegetables, to make burritos or a plate of nachos. This recipe keeps up to 5
days in the fridge. If it lasts that long . . .

1 tsp / 5 mL **extra virgin olive oil**
1 **onion—minced**
3 **cloves garlic**
1 19 oz / 540 mL can **black beans—drained and rinsed**
1 tbsp / 15 mL **chili powder**
1/2 cup / 125 mL **water**

1   Heat a large frying pan. Add the oil and the onion. Sauté
    for 1 minute, stirring constantly.

2   Add the garlic, black beans, chili powder and water.
    Simmer covered for 10 minutes.

3   Remove from heat. Purée using a hand-held blender,
    food processor or upright blender, or mash with a potato
    masher.

Serves 4

ONE SERVING	157 Calories
	9.3 g protein
	2.1 g fat
	9.4 g fiber
	136 mg sodium
	27 g carbohydrate
UHEP	1 Beans
	1/4 Fat

Burritos and Nachos

To make 4 burritos you'll need

4 small whole-wheat tortillas (see page 234)
1 recipe Refried Beans (see previous page)
2 tomatoes—chopped
1/2 cup / 125 mL **grated light Monterey Jack cheese**
2 cups / 500 mL shredded romaine lettuce
1 red pepper—diced
1 cup / 250 mL **salsa**

1   Spread 1/4 of the warm bean mixture over each tortilla. Top with tomatoes, cheese, lettuce, pepper and salsa. Roll to enclose filling.

ONE SERVING Burritos	337 Calories
	17.8 g protein
	6.4 g fat
	14.4 g fiber
	655 mg sodium
	53 g carbohydrate
UHEP	1 Beans
	1/4 Fat
	2 Vegetables & Fruit
	1 Grains
	1/4 Milk

To make nachos for two you'll need:

4 small whole-wheat tortillas (see page 234)
1/2 recipe **Refried Beans** (see previous page)
2 tomatoes
1/2 cup / 125 mL **light Monterey Jack Cheese**
1 red pepper—diced
1 cup / 250 mL **salsa**
1/4 cup / 50 mL **hot pickled peppers—diced**
1 green onion—diced

1   Cut each tortilla into 8 triangles. Place on a baking dish and bake for 5 to 7 minutes or until crisp at 400°F/200°C. Cool. Place them on a plate, top with refried beans, sprinkle with tomatoes, cheese, red pepper, salsa, pickled peppers and onion. Microwave for 1 minute on medium or until the cheese melts. Serve.

ONE SERVING Nachos	256 Calories
	12.7 g protein
	5.4 g fat
	9.3 g fiber
	412 mg sodium
	40 g carbohydrate
UHEP	1 Beans
	3 1/4 Vegetables & Fruit
	2 Grains
	1/2 Milk

6/10 - a bit boring

Amazing Black Bean Quesadillas

Kid-Approved

A big favorite at our house. During hockey season, when my son is busy at the rink, I double the recipe and keep the extra filling in the fridge for quick dinners before or after a game.

I have successfully demonstrated this recipe at countless cooking classes that I teach at the Loblaw's Cooking Schools in Toronto.

2 tsp / 10 mL **olive oil**
1 **onion—diced**
1 **red pepper—diced**
2 **cloves garlic—minced**
1/2 tsp / 2 mL **cumin**
1 19 oz / 540 mL can **black beans—drained and rinsed**
1 cup / 250 mL **salsa—mild, medium or spicy—your choice**
1 cup / 250 mL **grated light Monterey Jack cheese**
1/4 cup / 50 mL **cilantro—chopped—optional**
8 **small whole-wheat tortillas**

1   Heat the olive oil in a large frying pan. Add the onion and sauté for about 3 minutes or until soft.

2   Add the red pepper and the garlic. Sauté for 2 minutes.

3   Add the cumin, black beans and salsa, and stir well.

4   When the beans are heated through, remove from the heat.

5   Preheat the oven to 350°F/175°C. Put a baking sheet in the oven.

6   In a non-stick pan, place 1 tortilla shell. Spoon 1/4 of the bean mixture on top. Sprinkle with 1/4 of the cheese and 1/4 of the cilantro, if using. Place a tortilla shell on top. Brown one side and then very carefully flip it over to brown the other side. It helps if you place your hand on the top tortilla shell as you flip it over.

7   When cooked, place in the oven on the baking sheet. Cook remaining quesadillas.

8   When they are all cooked, cut each into quarters and serve with salsa and low-fat sour cream if desired.

Serves 4

KID-FRIENDLY TIP

Most little kids like the taste of mild salsa. My eleven-year-old likes medium, and most adults I know like spicy! What to do? Use the mildest one that your youngest likes and serve the other spicy salsa for dipping the quesadillas into.

WHERE DO I FIND WHOLE-WHEAT TORTILLAS?

They are usually in the bakery department, but sometimes you can find them in the Mexican Food Section. My favorite brand is Dempster's. It contains 100% whole wheat and no hydrogenated fats. I keep a package in my freezer for quick dinners like this quesadilla recipe and the Bean Burritos on page 233.

ONE SERVING	452 Calories
	22.7 g protein
	11.1 g fat
	13.1 g fiber
	589 mg sodium
	64 g carbohydrate
UHEP	1 Beans
	1 Vegetables & Fruit
	2 Grains
	1/2 Milk

Jerk Black Beans

TOO SPICY?

To make this dish a little less spicy add 3/4 cup/175 mL water instead of the 1/2 cup/125 mL.

KID-FRIENDLY TIP

Don't add the cayenne until after you have dished out what the kids are going to eat. Then either add the whole 1/4 tsp/1 mL cayenne, or half that amount according to taste, for the adults.

WHAT IS JERK?

A guy who says he'll call and never does. Oh, sorry, that is what is a jerk... Jerk is a Jamaican seasoning. The ingredients vary, depending on the cook, but usually include a blend of cinnamon, allspice, cloves, ginger, garlic, thyme and cayenne. It can be anywhere from extremely spicy to mild. This recipe is mild.

This isn't a really spicy version of jerk flavor. It is more like a "rookie" jerk flavor. If you want to turn up the heat add another 1/4 tsp/1 mL cayenne!

1 tbsp / 15 mL **olive oil**
1 1/2 tsp / 7 mL **thyme**
1 tsp / 5 mL **allspice**
1/4 tsp / 1 mL **cinnamon**
1/4 tsp / 1 mL **nutmeg**
1/4 tsp / 1 mL **cayenne**
1 **bunch green onions—chopped into 2-in/5-cm pieces, including the white part**
3 **cloves garlic—chopped**
1 19-oz / 540-mL can **black beans—drained and rinsed**
1/2 cup / 125 mL **water**

1 Heat a large frying pan. Add the olive oil, thyme, allspice, cinnamon, nutmeg and cayenne. Stir till the flavors hit you in the face! You'll know what that means when it happens!

2 Add the chopped green onions and garlic. Stir till coated with the spice mixture.

3 Add the black beans and the water.

4 Stir. Bring to the boil. Reduce heat to simmer. Cover and cook for 10 minutes.

5 Serve over brown rice.

Serves 4

ONE SERVING	167 Calories
	8.8 g protein
	4.1 g fat
	9.1 g fiber
	116 mg sodium
	25 g carbohydrate
UHEP	1 Beans
	3/4 Fat

South of the Border Lasagna

Kid-Approved

Okay, you have glanced down at the recipe and you saw that it had 16 steps!!! It's not as bad as it looks. Basically it's a recipe that involves stacking.

1 cup / 250 mL **light ricotta**
1 cup / 250 mL **grated light Monterey Jack cheese**
1 19-oz / 540-mL **can black beans—drained and rinsed**
1 tbsp / 15 mL **chili powder**
1 tsp / 5 mL **ground cumin**
3 **small whole-wheat tortillas** (see page 234)
1 cup / 250 mL **fresh or frozen corn**
1 cup / 250 mL **salsa—mild, medium or hot**
3 **large roasted red peppers** (see page 193)

1   Preheat the oven to 400°F/200°C.

2   In a medium bowl mix together the ricotta and 3/4 cup/175 mL of the Monterey Jack cheese. Reserve the remainder of the Monterey Jack cheese for later.

3   In a food processor grind the black beans, chili powder and cumin together. Don't purée the mixture. You want some of the beans to remain whole. If you don't have a food processor use a potato masher.

4   Begin the layering process.

5   Spray an 8-in/20-cm round casserole pan lightly with oil. Place one of the tortillas in the bottom.

6   Spoon ⅓ of the ricotta/Monterey Jack cheese mixture on top.

7   Spoon ⅓ of the bean mixture on top.

8   Spoon ⅓ of the corn on top.

9   Spoon ⅓ of the salsa on top.

10   And finally slice a red pepper in half and lay that on top of everything.

11   Repeat with the next tortilla shell. Press down lightly so that all those layers are compressed slightly.

12   Now put the next third of everything on in the same order.

13   Put the last tortilla shell on top and give it a light press.

14   Repeat the layering till you have used up all the ingredients and the only thing left is that leftover grated Monterey Jack cheese.

15   Sprinkle on the cheese and pop it into the oven. Bake for 40 minutes.

16   Here's the tricky part—you have to let it sit for 10 minutes before you cut it up or it will fall apart!

Serves 4

ONE SERVING	406 Calories
	27.4 g protein
	9.6 g fat
	12.2 g fiber
	484 mg sodium
	59 g carbohydrate
UHEP	1 Beans
	2 ½ Vegetables & Fruit
	¾ Grains
	1 Milk

Out-of-this-World Chili

Kid-Approved

There are as many chili recipes out there as there are pebbles on the beach. How poetic! The original recipe originated in Texas and had no beans in it at all. It was just a bowl of cooked meat with spices.

Well I'm sure this recipe would send any Texan worth their weight in beef for a loop. It doesn't have any meat in it at all—well nothing that originated on four legs. There is a meaty look to it, but it comes from Yves Veggie Ground Round, a soy meat-replacement. I've been using this in my chili for years and no one has ever figured it out. Don't be soy-challenged—give it a go.

ADULT VERSION

Want more spice? I usually add 1/4 tsp/1 mL red pepper flakes to the pot after I've served out my son's portion.

2 tbsp + 2 tsp / 40 mL **extra virgin olive oil**
1 **onion—diced**
1 **carrot—diced**
1 **red pepper—diced**
3 **cloves garlic—minced**
1 19 oz / 540 mL can **black beans—drained and rinsed**
1 19 oz / 540 mL can **kidney beans—drained and rinsed**
1 28 oz / 796 mL can **plum tomatoes**
2 tbsp / 25 mL **tomato paste**
1/4 cup / 50 mL **medium salsa**
2 tbsp + 1 tsp / 35 mL **chili powder**
1 tsp / 5 mL **cumin**
1 tsp / 5 mL **oregano**
1 tsp / 5 mL **basil**
1 12 oz / 340 g pkg **Yves Veggie Ground Round**

1   Heat a large pot. Add the oil and onion. Sauté till the onion is translucent, approx. 3 minutes.

2   Add the carrot, red pepper and garlic. Sauté for 2 minutes.

3   Add the black beans, kidney beans, plum tomatoes, tomato paste, salsa, chili powder, cumin, oregano and basil.

4   Bring to the boil. Reduce heat, cover and simmer for 20 minutes or until the carrot is cooked.

5   Add the package of Yves Veggie Ground Round and heat through. Serve.

Serves 8

ONE SERVING	248 Calories
	15.8 g protein
	5 g fat
	13 g fiber
	608 mg sodium
	36 g carbohydrate
UHEP	1 Beans
	1 Fat
	1 Vegetables & Fruit
	3/4 Soy

Mexican Lentil Casserole

Totally Kid-Approved

FEELING EXPERIMENTAL?

It also tastes great with kidney beans or black beans instead of the lentils.

Remember that hunky prof I mentioned in the Mairlyn's World Famous Beans and Rice blurb? Well he suggested that our nutrition class attend a vegetarian seminar on cooking with beans and lentils. I signed up, still hoping that this was more like a "Fountain of Youth Seminar" or "How to Look Young Forever" class. I looked the same when I left, but I did leave with some fabulous ideas for recipes. This was one of them.

1 tbsp + 1 tsp / 20 mL **extra virgin olive oil**
1 **large onion—chopped**
6 **cloves garlic—minced**
1 **large red pepper—diced**
1 **orange pepper—diced**
1/2 tsp / 2 mL **red pepper flakes**
2 tsp / 10 mL **cumin**
1 tsp / 5 mL **coriander**
1 tsp / 5 mL **oregano**
1 28 oz / 796 mL can **whole plum tomatoes**
1 19 oz / 540 mL can **lentils—drained and rinsed**
1 cup / 250 mL **grated light old cheddar**

Topping
3/4 cup / 175 mL **cornmeal**
1/4 tsp / 1 mL **salt**
1 tsp / 5 mL **baking powder**
1/4 tsp / 1 mL **baking soda**
1 **omega-3 egg**
1/2 cup / 125 mL **buttermilk**

ONE SERVING	281 Calories
	15.7 g protein
	8.7 g fat
	7.6 g fiber
	780 mg sodium
	37 g carbohydrate
UHEP	3/4 Beans
	3/4 Fat
	1 1/2 Vegetables & Fruit
	1/2 Milk

1   Preheat the oven to 375°F/190°C. Lightly spray a 9 x 13-in/23 x 33-cm pan. Set aside.

2   Heat a large frying pan and add the olive oil and onion. Sauté for 1 minute.

3   Add the garlic, red pepper, orange pepper, red pepper flakes, cumin, coriander and oregano. Sauté for 2 minutes.

4   Add the plum tomatoes and the lentils. Bring to the boil.

5   Pour into the prepared pan. Top with the grated cheese.

6   In a small bowl mix together the topping ingredients. Stir well. Spoon over the cheese.

7   Bake for 25 minutes.

Serves 4

8/10 — too spicey (I think our chilli powder is hightest).

Taco-Taco Salad

Totally Kid-Approved

Andrew and I were at a fast-food place and he ordered the Taco Salad. He loved it. Midbite he said, "Hey, Mom, you should make this for your new book." Well, I took his advice and here it is. A totally kid-approved fast meal, ready in 20 minutes, that gets gobbled up every time you serve it.

4 **small whole-wheat tortillas** (see page 234)
1 tbsp + 1 tsp / 20 mL **extra virgin olive oil**
1 **medium onion—chopped**
2 **cloves garlic—minced**
7 oz / 200 g **extra lean ground turkey**
1 tbsp / 15 mL **chili powder**
1 tsp / 5 mL **cumin**
1/2 tsp / 2 mL **oregano**
1/4 cup / 50 mL **tomato paste**
1 cup / 250 mL **water**
2 tbsp / 25 mL **ketchup**
1 tsp / 5 mL **Worcestershire sauce**
1 19-oz / 540-mL **can black beans—drained and rinsed**
1 **head of romaine**
1 **red pepper**

1   Preheat the oven to 400°F/200°C. Cut each tortilla into 4 pieces. Place on a cookie sheet and put into the oven. Bake for 5 to 7 minutes until lightly browned. Let cool on the cookie sheet while you prepare the rest of the recipe.

2   Meanwhile, heat the oil in a large frying pan over medium-high heat.

3   Add the onions and sauté till almost cooked, 3 to 5 minutes.

4   Add the garlic and continue sautéing for 1 minute.

5   Add the ground turkey and brown.

6   Add the chili powder, cumin and oregano. Stir well.

7   Add the tomato paste, water, ketchup and Worcestershire sauce. Stir well.

8   Stir in the beans and lower heat to medium. Heat through. This will take about 3 to 5 minutes.

9   While you wait, wash and then chop up the romaine and red pepper into bite-sized pieces. Divide the lettuce equally among the 4 plates.

10   When the bean mixture is hot, remove from the heat and spoon 1/4 of the mixture over the lettuce. Sprinkle with the red pepper. Serve with the baked tortillas. Watch your kids gobble this up! Yeah! Something they like!!! Make a mental note to serve this at least once a week till they move out.

Serves 4

ONE SERVING with tortillas	369 Calories 22.6 g protein 11.3 g fat 12.5 g fiber 500 mg sodium 49 g carbohydrate
UHEP	1 Beans 1 Fat 1 3/4 Vegetables & Fruit 1 Grains 1/2 Meat
ONE SERVING without tortillas	274 Calories 19.9 g protein 9.3 g fat 10.8 g fiber 358 mg sodium 34 g carbohydrate
UHEP	1 Beans 1 Fat 1 3/4 Vegetables & Fruit 1/2 Meat

Jazzy Beans

Kid-Approved

Okay, you've just walked in the door, you are so hungry that you may pass out at any minute, and for some strange reason, you're crabby! All you have in the house is a can of beans, an onion, 1 red pepper, ketchup, mustard and molasses. Sound like your life? Hey, it's mine!

Whatever you do, don't use the beans made with maple syrup or molasses; this will be too sweet. I use plain old baked beans with tomato sauce from Heinz.

1 tbsp + 1 tsp / 20 mL **extra virgin olive oil**
1 **onion—chopped**
1 **red pepper—diced**
1 14-oz / 398-mL can **beans in tomato sauce**
2 tbsp / 25 mL **ketchup**
1 tbsp / 15 mL **Dijon mustard**
1 tbsp / 15 mL **molasses**

1 Heat a medium pan. Add the oil, onion and red pepper. Sauté for 3 minutes.

2 Add remaining ingredients. Simmer covered for 10 minutes.

Serves 4

SERVING TIP
Goes well with steamed broccoli or if you really do have nothing in the house, hopefully you at least have frozen peas! Always great to have on hand.

ONE SERVING	209 Calories
	7.7 g protein
	5.5 g fat
	7.1 g fiber
	502 mg sodium
	33 g carbohydrate
UHEP	1 Beans
	1 Fat

So Soya+ Stir-Fry

You've probably seen the box of So Soya+ slices in the produce section of your grocery store and wondered what the heck they were. Well, here's your chance to broaden your taste horizons. They are little nuggets of soy flour that need to be reconstituted with a hot liquid. They basically take on the flavor of whatever the liquid is, and voilà, a soy serving. We eat this stir-fry once a week. Andrew thinks it's chicken…okay, I told him it was chicken…okay, I sort of fibbed. But it's a healthy fib.

2 cups / 500 mL **chicken stock or lower-sodium chicken stock**
2 tbsp / 25 mL **oyster sauce** (see page 174)
4 **cloves garlic—minced**
1 tbsp / 15 mL **coarsely grated ginger**
1 1/3 cups / 325 mL **So Soya+**
2 cups / 500 mL **broccoli florets**
2 cups / 500 mL **cauliflower florets**
1 cup / 250 mL **carrots**
2 **green onions**
1 tbsp / 15 mL **cornstarch**
1 tbsp + 1 tsp / 20 mL **extra virgin olive oil**

1   Put the chicken stock, oyster sauce, minced garlic and ginger into a large pot and bring to the boil. Add the So Soya+. Stir in, reduce heat and simmer, stirring occasionally for 20 minutes.

2   While it is simmering, chop up the broccoli and cauliflower. Slice the carrots into 1/2-in/1.2-cm slices.

3   Chop the green onions into 3-in/7.5-cm pieces.

4   When the So Soya+ slices are done, drain the liquid and reserve. Add the cornstarch to the liquid. Set aside.

5   Heat a large frying pan or wok. Add the oil. Toss in the broccoli, cauliflower and carrots. Stir often.

6   Add the So Soya+. Stir. Heat through. Add the green onions.

7   Stir in the cornstarch liquid. Stir till it becomes clear and bubbles.

8   Serve. Tell everyone that it's chicken. See what happens!

Serves 4

ONE SERVING	141 Calories
	12.4 g protein
	5.1 g fat
	6.6 g fiber
	578 mg sodium
	16 g carbohydrate
lower-sodium chicken stock	392 mg sodium
UHEP	1 Fat
	2 1/2 Vegetables & Fruit
	1 Soy

Fruit

CHOCOLATE SOY MILK

All chocolate soy milks do not taste alike. Experiment, try them all. Our two family favorites are So Nice and So Good.

FROZEN BANANA?

Cut overripe bananas into 2-in/ 5 cm chunks and freeze them. When the blender drink urge hits you—break off 6 to 8 chunks, and voilà, the right amount that equals 1 banana.

Here is a series of blender shakes. The shakes are thick like a milkshake without the ice cream, and sometimes even without the milk! The trick is to use frozen fruit. As the frozen banana, strawberries, or raspberries are puréed into the milk or soy milk they freeze the rest of the ingredients, giving you a rich creamy drink.

Super Chocolate Banana Soy Shake

With the Super Chocolate Banana Soy Shake get your soy and chocolate fix all at the same time.

1 cup / 250 mL **chocolate soy milk**
1 **frozen banana—chunks**

1   Whirl everything in a blender. Drink!

Serves 1

ONE SERVING	227 Calories
	7.5 g protein
	3.6 g fat
	2.8 g fiber
	141 mg sodium
	45 g carbohydrate
UHEP	2 Vegetables & Fruit
	1 Soy

Super Chocolate Banana Tofu Milkshake

Still a little tofu-challenged? Well this version in my series of quick blender drinks includes silken tofu, and no you can't taste it! Get your soy for the day. Give it a whirl, literally!

1/2 cup / 125 mL **skim milk**
1 **frozen banana—cut into chunks**
1/2 cup / 125 mL **silken tofu**
2 tbsp / 25 mL **chocolate syrup**

1 Whirl everything together in a blender. Drink.

Serves 1

Super Berry Shake

Another tofu recipe to drink.

1/2 cup / 125 mL **skim milk**
1 cup / 250 mL **frozen strawberries—about 8 strawberries**
or 1 cup/250 mL **frozen raspberries**
1/2 cup / 125 mL **silken tofu**
2 tbsp / 25 mL **honey**

1 Whirl everything together in the blender. Drink.

Serves 1

WHAT THE HECK IS SILKEN TOFU?
Tofu comes in many different styles and textures. Silken tofu has a very smooth texture—like silk! It is perfect in blender drinks, and no, you won't be able to taste it! Tofu is such a chameleon. Using strawberries? It will taste like strawberries. Using raspberries? You guessed it—tastes like raspberries, etc...

ONE SERVING Super Chocolate Banana Tofu Milkshake	315 Calories
	11.5 g protein
	4.6 g fat
	3.5 g fiber
	29 mg sodium
	60 g carbohydrate
UHEP	2 Vegetables & Fruit
	1/2 Milk
	1 Soy

ONE SERVING Super Berry Shake	257 Calories
	10.6 g protein
	3.7 g fat
	2.3 g fiber
	3 mg sodium
	49 g carbohydrate
UHEP	2 Vegetables & Fruit
	1/2 Milk
	1 Soy

Soy Milk Fruit Smoothies

FROZEN BERRIES
In berry season, I freeze my own. In the off season I buy unsweetened frozen berries in the freezer case at my local grocery store. Either way they are great—it's your choice.

ONE SERVING	187 Calories
	9.3 g protein
Super Soy Strawberry Smoothie	5.0 g fat
	1.8 g fiber
	158 mg sodium
	26 g carbohydrate
UHEP	1 Vegetables & Fruit
	1 Soy

ONE SERVING	233 Calories
	9.23 g protein
Big Blue Berry Purple Smoothie	5.4 g fat
	2.94 g fiber
	141 mg sodium
	40 g carbohydrate
UHEP	1 Vegetables & Fruit
	1 Soy

Super Soy Strawberry Smoothie

What an alliteration—four S's!!!—which is also superb! That makes it five! No frozen strawberries? Use frozen raspberries.

1 cup / 250 mL **strawberry soy milk**
1/2 cup / 125 mL **frozen strawberries—about 4**

1 Whirl everything together in the blender. Drink.

Serves 1

Big Blue Berry Purple Smoothie

1 cup / 250 mL **vanilla soy milk**
3/4 cup / 175 mL **frozen blueberries**

1 Whirl everything together in the blender. Drink.

Serves 1

Strawberries with French Vanilla Yogurt

I first started eating this when I joined Weight Watchers in the 1980s. Back then I used plain yogurt, but now my favorite is French Vanilla. The brand that I like the best is Astro's Biobest line. It's low in fat, high in flavor, and has two active bacterial cultures that are important for a healthy intestine.

1/2 cup / 125 mL **low-fat French Vanilla yogurt**
2 tbsp / 25 mL **orange juice concentrate** (see page 165)
1 cup / 250 mL **sliced strawberries—about 8**

1   Mix together the yogurt and the orange juice concentrate. Pour over the sliced strawberries. Eat!

Serves 1

ONE SERVING	115 Calories
	6.6 g protein
	1.3 g fat
	2.4 g fiber
	81 g sodium
	30 g carbohydrate
UHEP	2 Vegetables & Fruit
	1/4 Milk

Dried Fruit Compote

In the dead of an Ontario winter when fresh fruit means either apples, oranges or bananas, this is a great dish to make. Have it at breakfast, as a snack, or over low-fat frozen yogurt as a dessert.

1 1/2 cups / 375 mL **orange juice**
16 **prunes**
16 **dried apricots**
1/3 cup / 75 mL **dried cranberries**
1 **cinnamon stick**

1   In a medium pot mix all the ingredients together.

2   Bring to the boil. Cover, reduce the heat to low and simmer for 10 minutes.

3   Cool. Store in the fridge for up to 1 week.

Serves 4

ONE SERVING	216 Calories
	2.1 g protein
	0.4 g fat
	4.4 g fiber
	18 mg sodium
	54 g carbohydrate
UHEP	3 Vegetables & Fruit

Frozen Raspberry Yogurt

When it comes to frozen yogurt, give me raspberry!
This is such a cinch to make, and tastes so decadent,
you won't believe that it has only two ingredients and
takes 3 minutes to make! You do, however, need a
food processor or a blender.

2 cups / 500 mL **frozen unsweetened raspberries**
1 cup / 250 mL **low-fat French Vanilla yogurt**

1   Put the frozen raspberries and the yogurt into the bowl
    of a food processor or a blender. Put on the lid and
    blend till smooth. This makes a rather loud noise, but
    don't worry, your food processor or blender can handle
    it. Serve!

2   Too easy, eh?

Serves 4

ONE SERVING	106 Calories
	4.1 g protein
	0.8 g fat
	1.3 g fiber
	40 mg sodium
	21 g carbohydrate
UHEP	1 Vegetables & Fruit
	1/4 Milk

Blueberry Nectarine Crisp

SERVING TIP

This tastes great over some low-fat ice cream or low-fat yogurt.

COOKING TIP

If using frozen fruit bake for 50 to 55 minutes.

This blueberry crisp is not too sweet and is great to serve after a light, summer dinner. If blueberries and peaches are out of season, you can always buy frozen ones. I use the tiny wild blueberries that I can buy during July and August here in Ontario, then freeze them myself for the winter.

3 cups / 750 mL **wild blueberries**
3 **peaches or nectarines**
3 tbsp / 45 mL **honey**
1/2 tsp / 2 mL **cinnamon**
2 tbsp / 25 mL **whole-wheat flour**

Topping
1 cup / 250 mL **old-fashioned rolled oats**
1/4 cup / 50 mL **whole-wheat flour**
1/2 cup / 125 mL **brown sugar**
2 tsp / 10 mL **cinnamon**
1/4 cup / 50 mL **canola oil**

1 Preheat the oven to 350°F/175°C.

2 Wash the blueberries. Peel the peaches or nectarines and slice thinly. Add the honey, cinnamon and the 2 tbsp/ 25 mL of whole-wheat flour. Mix together in a bowl. Pour into a lightly greased 8 x 8-in/20 x 20-cm pan.

3 Mix the topping ingredients together with a fork. Blend until the ingredients look wet. Sprinkle over the fruit. Lightly press down.

4 Bake for 35 to 40 minutes. Let cool. Serve.

Serves 8

ONE SERVING	244 Calories
	3.2 g protein
	8.0 g fat
	4.2 g fiber
	8 mg sodium
	44 g carbohydrate
UHEP	1 1/2 Fat
	1 1/2 Vegetables & Fruit
	1/4 Grains

Muffins, Pancakes and French Toast

GROUND FLAXSEED

I like to buy flaxseed whole and then grind them up in my coffee bean mill. That way I only grind up what I will be using in the next week. Don't become overzealous and grind them into flour. Just keep pulsing until they look like coarse sand. Once the flaxseed have been ground, store them in a covered container in the fridge. A coffee bean mill is the only thing that grinds up the seeds well enough. Trust me; I have tried blenders, food processors, an old fashioned coffee bean grinder and a hammer! The coffee bean mill works the best. You can also buy flaxseed already ground. It will be in the refrigerated section in the store. That's the big tip-off; you need to store it in your fridge.

WHAT IS BUTTERMILK?

A lot of people think that buttermilk is really high in fat and therefore bad for you. Wrong! In the old farm days buttermilk was the liquid left over after butter was made, hence the name. Today it is made by adding a special bacteria to nonfat or low-fat milk, giving it a slightly thickened consistency and a tangy flavor.

I use it a lot in low-fat cooking. I find that it adds lots of flavor to muffins and other quickbreads. So if you bought the buttermilk just for this recipe, look through the other muffin recipes. You can use it for those ones too.

ONE MUFFIN	190 Calories
	5.2 g protein
	5.8 g fat
	6.0 g fiber
	217 mg sodium
	31 g carbohydrate
UHEP	1 Flax
	1/2 Vegetables & Fruit
	1 1/2 Grains

Banana Chocolate Chip Muffins

Totally Kid-Approved!

Yummy!!! These muffins are my son's favorite. He can eat them for breakfast, lunch, snacks, or even as a dessert, but not all in the same day! They are loaded with fiber as well as flavor. They taste too good to be "good for you!" For a really moist muffin make sure that the bananas are really ripe. Think of overripe bananas, think of a too-ripe banana to eat as a snack, think that the skin is so black that they look a little too ripe to even think about eating. These are the perfect ones for recipes like this.

Dry Ingredients
1 cup / 250 mL **whole-wheat flour**
3/4 cup / 175 mL **wheat bran**
3/4 cup / 175 mL **ground flaxseed**
1/4 cup / 50 mL **mini chocolate chips**
1 tbsp / 15 mL **baking powder**
1 tsp / 5 mL **baking soda**
1 tsp / 5 mL **cinnamon**

Wet Ingredients
1 1/2 cups / 375 mL **mashed banana, approx. 4–5 really ripe bananas**
3/4 cup / 175 mL **dark brown sugar**
3/4 cup / 175 mL **buttermilk**
1 **omega-3 egg**

1 Preheat the oven to 400°F/200°C.

2 Line a muffin tin with large paper cup liners.

3 In a large bowl mix together all the dry ingredients using a fork or a wire whisk.

4 In a medium bowl beat together all the wet ingredients. The mashed banana really needs to be mixed in well.

5 Pour the wet ingredients into the dry ingredients and mix till just combined.

6 Spoon into muffin cups and bake for 20 to 25 minutes or until done.

Makes 12

Super Nutritious Chocolate Chip Bran Muffins

These muffins are loaded with powerfully nutritious ingredients like whole grains, flaxseed, prunes and buttermilk.

Warning—they taste great! So great that you may be inclined to eat 3 or 4 at one sitting. Don't. The thank you note from your colon will be more than you expected.

Dry Ingredients

1 1/4 cups / 300 mL **whole-wheat flour**
1 cup / 250 mL **wheat bran**
3/4 cup / 175 mL **ground flaxseed** (see previous page)
1/2 cup / 125 mL **chopped dates**
1/4 cup / 50 mL **mini chocolate chips**
1 tbsp / 15 mL **cinnamon**
1 tsp / 5 mL **baking powder**
1 tsp / 5 mL **baking soda**

Wet Ingredients

1 1/4 cups / 300 mL **buttermilk** (see previous page)
1 **omega-3 egg**
1 4 1/2-oz / 128-mL jar **strained prunes—no added sugar or starch**
3/4 cup / 175 mL **dark brown sugar**
1/4 cup / 50 mL **molasses**

1 Preheat the oven to 400°F/200°C.

2 Line a muffin tin with large paper cup liners.

3 In a large bowl mix together all the dry ingredients using a fork or a wire whisk.

4 In a medium bowl beat together all the wet ingredients.

5 Pour the wet ingredients into the dry ingredients and mix till just combined.

6 Spoon into muffin cups and bake for 20 to 25 minutes or until done.

Makes 12

DO YOU REMEMBER THE MUFFIN METHOD FROM GRADE 8 HOME EC?

Mix all the dry ingredients in one bowl. Mix all the wet ingredients in another bowl. Add the wet to the dry and stir until just mixed. Okay, so you're probably thinking, brown sugar is not a wet ingredient. Well, you would be correct! You are not the "Weakest Link," go straight to the top of the class, your Home Ec. teacher would be proud. It isn't a wet ingredient, but it does combine for a better muffin when dissolved with the other wet ingredients. Just call this the Mairlyn Muffin Method.

A JAR OF STRAINED PRUNES!

Where the heck are the jars of strained prunes in the maze they call the supermarket? Try the baby food section. Make sure that you buy the type that has no sugar or starch added.

WHAT DOES "OR UNTIL DONE" MEAN?

It's the toothpick test. Insert a toothpick into the center of the muffin; if it comes out clean the muffin is done.

BAKING TIP: FOR ALL THE MUFFIN RECIPES

You can substitute equal amounts of soy milk for buttermilk; just add 2 tsp/10 mL of lemon juice to the soy milk to sour it.

ONE MUFFIN	234 Calories
	6.2 g protein
	6.0 g fat
	7.7 g fiber
	169 mg sodium
	41 g carbohydrate
UHEP	1 Flax
	1 1/2 Grains

Pumpkin Chocolate Chip Muffins

Kid-Approved

Another high-fiber/low-fat muffin. This one combines the high fiber of All-Bran Buds cereal with the excellent nutrition from pumpkin, with just enough mini chocolate chips to add a little decadence to the whole thing.

Dry Ingredients

1 1/4 cups / 300 mL **whole-wheat flour**
1/2 cup / 125 mL **wheat bran**
3/4 cup / 175 mL **ground flaxseed**
2 tbsp / 25 mL **wheat germ**
1 tbsp / 15 mL **cinnamon**
1 tbsp / 15 mL **baking powder**
1 tsp / 5 mL **baking soda**
1/4 cup / 50 mL **mini chocolate chips**

Wet Ingredients

1 cup / 250 mL **buttermilk**
1 cup / 250 mL **pumpkin purée**
1 cup / 250 mL **dark brown sugar**
1 **omega-3 egg**
1/2 cup / 125 mL **All-Bran Buds cereal**

1   Preheat the oven to 400°F/200°C.

2   Line a muffin tin with large paper cup liners.

3   In a large bowl mix together all the dry ingredients using a fork or a wire whisk.

4   In a medium bowl beat together all the wet ingredients.

5   Pour the wet ingredients into the dry ingredients and mix till just combined.

6   Spoon into muffin cups and bake for 20 to 25 minutes or until done.

Makes 12

ONE MUFFIN	210 Calories
	6.3 g protein
	6.0 g fat
	8.0 g fiber
	250 mg sodium
	36 g carbohydrate
UHEP	1 Flax
	1 1/2 Grains

Blueberry Muffins

Kid-Approved

A great way to get those blueberries into your diet. These muffins are delicious right out of the oven or up to 3 days later. Double the recipe and freeze 1 or 2 muffins in small baggies. When packing lunches for school or the office pop a frozen package into your lunch bag. They'll be thawed out by lunch, making you the envy of all who work with you. You could be nice and pack extras for the office . . . or just tell everyone to buy this book! (Subliminal advertising.)

Dry Ingredients
1 cup / 250 mL **whole-wheat flour**
1/2 cup / 125 mL **wheat bran**
1 tbsp / 15 mL **baking powder**
1 tsp / 5 mL **baking soda**
2 tsp / 10 mL **cinnamon**
1 1/2 cups / 375 mL **fresh or frozen blueberries**

Wet Ingredients
1 **omega-3 egg**
1/4 cup / 50 mL **canola oil**
1 cup / 250 mL **1% yogurt**
1 cup / 250 mL **oat bran**
3/4 cup / 175 mL **white sugar**
2 tbsp / 25 mL **orange marmalade**

1 Preheat the oven to 400°F/200°C.

2 Line a muffin tin with large paper cup liners.

3 In a medium bowl mix together all the wet ingredients. Set aside while you measure out the dry ingredients. This will give the oat bran a chance to absorb most of the liquid. A little tip that will help make you a culinary wizard!

4 In a large bowl mix together all the dry ingredients using a fork or a wire whisk.

5 Pour the wet ingredients into the dry ingredients and mix till just combined. Gently fold in the blueberries. Don't overmix or you will have purple muffins. This isn't a bad thing, just a weird thing.

6 Spoon into muffin cups and bake for 20 to 25 minutes or until done.

Makes 12

SHOULD I USE FRESH OR FROZEN BLUEBERRIES?

It really doesn't matter which you choose. I use frozen blueberries when they are out of season and fresh ones when they are in season. In August I freeze the fresh wild ones so that I am all stocked up for the winter.

Wild blueberries are tinier than the commercial ones and I like the way they bake up better. If you do go with the frozen ones don't worry that the batter is really thick. The berries are freezing it! They will bake the same. Just make sure that you test for doneness. And that would be? Using a toothpick to see if it comes out clean. If it's not all gummy with raw batter the muffins are done.

ONE MUFFIN	201 Calories
	4.8 g protein
	6.3 g fat
	4.5 g fiber
	211 mg sodium
	32 g carbohydrate
UHEP	1 Fat
	1/4 Vegetables & Fruit
	1 1/2 Grains

Cranberry Orange Muffins

WHERE DO I FIND DRIED CRANBERRIES?

If you have a bulk section in your store they are usually with all the other dried fruits. If not, most grocery stores carry them in the produce department for some unknown reason. They are packaged by Oceanspray and are called Craisins.

KID-FRIENDLY TIP

Make the Banana Chocolate Chip Muffins. You eat the Cranberry Orange, they eat the Banana Chocolate Chip. It's a win-win situation. Or better yet, teach them how to make the Banana Chocolate Chip Muffins themselves!

ONE MUFFIN	230 Calories
	6.17 g protein
	6.5 g fat
	6.7 g fiber
	188 mg sodium
	41 g carbohydrate
UHEP	1 Flax
	1/4 Vegetables & Fruit
	1 Grains

I love cranberries! My Fairy Godmother, Nina, used to make cranberry walnut tarts every Christmas for me. They were her specialty. Right after I put up my Christmas tree she would send them over but she stopped making them the year she moved into a retirement home. I eventually forgot about them until this year when she gave me the recipe. My mouth watered as I read over the ingredients. Well, tarts are a fat "no-no," so I came up with a healthy-fat "yes-yes" variation! Thanks, Nina.

Dry Ingredients
1 cup / 250 mL **whole-wheat flour**
1/2 cup / 125 mL **wheat bran**
3/4 cup / 175 mL **ground flaxseed**
1/4 cup / 50 mL **walnuts—coarsely chopped**
1 tbsp / 15 mL **baking powder**
1 tsp / 5 mL **baking soda**
1 tsp / 5 mL **cinnamon**
2/3 cup / 150 mL **dried cranberries**
1 cup / 250 mL **fresh or frozen whole cranberries**
1 **orange—zest of**

Wet Ingredients
1 **omega-3 egg**
1 cup / 250 mL **buttermilk**
1 1/4 cups / 300 mL **dark brown sugar**
2/3 cup / 150 mL **oat bran**

1   Preheat the oven to 400°F/200°C.

2   Line a muffin tin with large paper cup liners.

3   In a large bowl mix together the whole-wheat flour, wheat bran, ground flaxseed, walnuts, baking powder, baking soda and cinnamon.

4   Add the dried cranberries, whole cranberries and zest from the orange.

5   In a medium bowl mix together all the wet ingredients.

6   Add the wet ingredients to the dry ingredients and mix until just combined.

7   Spoon into muffin cups. Bake for 20 to 25 minutes or until done.

8   Eat the zested orange while the muffins are baking! It counts as 1 fruit serving! Every little bit helps.

Makes 12

Apple and Oat Pancakes

Totally Kid-Approved

When I was a kid my dad would make pancakes on the weekends. I can still see him in my mind's eye—getting out the old frying pan that didn't have a handle, setting out the ingredients, the batter hitting the pan and then the smell of pancakes and maple syrup wafting around the kitchen.

I still make pancakes on the weekend. I love the memory connection and the tradition that I am passing on to my son.

1 1/2 cups / 375 mL **1% yogurt—I prefer Astro's Biobest**
3/4 cup / 175 mL **quick rolled oats**
1/2 cup / 125 mL **skim milk**
1 **omega-3 egg**
1 tbsp / 15 mL **maple syrup or brown sugar**
2 **apples—peeled**
1 cup / 250 mL **whole-wheat flour**
1/4 cup / 50 mL **ground flaxseed**
2 tsp / 10 mL **cinnamon**
1 tsp / 5 mL **baking soda**
1 tsp / 5 mL **baking powder**
2 cups / 500 mL **applesauce—optional**

1   In a large bowl mix together the yogurt, quick oats, skim milk, egg and maple syrup. Grate the peeled apple right into the bowl.

2   Measure out the whole-wheat flour, flaxseed, cinnamon, baking soda and baking powder right into the large bowl. Mix it all together well. You can't overmix this recipe!

3   Heat a large non-stick skillet to medium high heat. Spray with a little oil.

4   Pour out the batter so that you end up with 16 pancakes in all. These pancakes are very light, so be careful when you flip them over. Keep the cooked ones in the oven at 250°F/120°C to stay warm.

5   Serve each pancake with 1 tbsp/15 mL of applesauce overtop, then top with a little pure maple syrup!

Makes 16. Serves 4.

PURE MAPLE SYRUP VS FAKE MAPLE SYRUP: THE GREAT TREE DEBATE

This has been a question plaguing Canadians for years: tree syrup or nontree syrup? Once you've watched the golden elixir of the Mighty Maple Tree slowly dripping its way down the side of a stack of fluffy pancakes on a cold winter morning with the sound of loons calling on the wind in the background and the soft flakes of snow floating down on the frosted windowpane, then that first mouthful, the sensuous flavor enticing you for yet another mouthful, wanting you to go on and on and on . . . oh, heck, you never go back to any substitute.

ONE SERVING 4 pancakes	339 Calories
	15.1 g protein
	7.5 g fat
	9.4 g fiber
	474 mg sodium
	58 g carbohydrate
UHEP	1 Flax
	1/2 Vegetables & Fruit
	3 Grains
	1/2 Milk
ONE SERVING 4 pancakes with applesauce	395 Calories
	15.3 g protein
	7.8 g fat
	11.7 g fiber
	486 mg sodium
	72 g carbohydrate
UHEP	1 Flax
	1 1/2 Vegetables & Fruit
	3 Grains
	1/2 Milk

Whole-Wheat Blueberry Buttermilk Pancakes

Totally Kid-Approved

NO BLUEBERRIES?

Liz says it's okay to use mini chocolate chips instead, but just 1/4 cup/50 mL.

I made these pancakes for my son's class on Shrove Tuesday last year. Twenty-five 10–11-year-olds representing seven different countries gobbled them up, and asked for more. That meets the criteria for totally kid-approved. One little girl even asked if I could make some more to send home to her parents!

Dry Ingredients
1 cup / 250 mL **whole-wheat flour**
1/2 cup / 125 mL **wheat germ**
1 tbsp / 15 mL **white sugar**
1 tsp / 5 mL **baking soda**
1 tsp / 5 mL **baking powder**
1 tbsp / 15 mL **cinnamon**

Wet Ingredients
1 **large omega-3 egg**
1 tbsp + 1 tsp / 20 mL **canola oil**
1 1/2 cups / 375 mL **buttermilk**
1 cup / 250 mL **blueberries**

ONE SERVING 4 pancakes	303 Calories
	14.0 g protein
	8.9 g fat
	7.8 g fiber
	505 mg sodium
	44 g carbohydrate

UHEP	1 Fat
	1/2 Vegetables & Fruit
	3 Grains
	1/4 Milk

1   In a large bowl measure out all the dry ingredients. Mix them together using a fork or a wire whisk.

2   In a medium bowl mix together the egg, canola oil and buttermilk.

3   Pour this into the dry ingredients and stir till just mixed. Add the blueberries and stir in gently.

4   Heat a large non-stick skillet. Spray with a little oil.

5   Pour out the batter so that you end up with 16 pancakes in all. Keep the cooked ones in the oven at 250°F/120°C to stay warm.

6   Serve with real maple syrup.

Makes 16. Serves 4.

French Toast

Totally Kid-Approved

This was one of the first things that I taught my son to cook. It requires following directions, measuring, beating, cooking over heat and using the oven! Once a Home Ec. teacher, always a Home Ec. teacher!

Well, aside from Andrew gaining confidence in the kitchen, I've also guaranteed myself a great "breakfast in bed" on Mother's Day and my birthday! One year I even got scrambled eggs as well. Whoever Andrew decides to spend his life with, I want a thank-you note.

4 **omega-3 eggs**
1 cup / 250 mL **skim milk or soy milk**
2 tsp / 10 mL **cinnamon**
1 tsp / 5 mL **pure vanilla extract—optional**
8 **slices whole-wheat bread**

1   In a shallow bowl beat together the eggs, skim milk or soy milk, cinnamon and vanilla, if using.

2   Heat a large non-stick frying pan. Turn on the oven to 200°F/95°C.

3   Soak the bread in the egg mixture, one slice at a time.

4   Lightly spray the pan with canola oil. Cook each slice of bread over medium heat till done on both sides. Keep the "done ones" in the oven till all the slices are cooked.

5   Serve with maple syrup, light or regular.

Serves 4

WHICH ONE DO I USE? SKIM MILK OR SOY MILK?

Well, the choice is up to you. If you are trying to add soy to your diet, this recipe is great. You won't be able to tell the difference between the French toast made with milk or the soy milk. My eleven-year-old's best friend, who is a really picky eater, couldn't tell. And if Andrew D. can't tell, no one can.

WHOLE-WHEAT BREAD

Family whole-wheat-challenged? Once again I find that this recipe is a great way to introduce a new ingredient. Whole-wheat, aside from being one of the wonderful whole-grain foods Liz talks about in the Wonderful Whole Grains chapter, has more flavor than white, and even my son's whole-wheat challenged friend gobbles it up when I serve it at my house.

PURE VANILLA EXTRACT

If you don't have the pure stuff, don't even think of using the artificial. Back away from the cupboard. Write a note to buy some of the real thing the next time you are out shopping. And throw out that fake stuff!

ONE SERVING	226 Calories
	12.2 g protein
	8.9 g fat
	5.6 g fiber
	210 mg sodium
	27 g carbohydrate
UHEP	1 Egg
	2 Grains
	1/4 Milk

Cookies, Loaves, Treats and Cake

10/10

Chocolate Chip Cookies

Totally Kid-Approved

Hey! I thought that cookies were on the no-no list! Well everyone needs a cookie once and a while and of course this book *had* to have chocolate chip cookies.

These are the crunchy kind of chocolate chip cookies that I like the best. If you want a chewier cookie omit 1/4 cup/50 mL of the flour and bake for only 8 to 10 minutes.

1/2 cup / 125 mL **nonhydrogenated margarine**
1/2 cup / 125 mL **brown sugar**
1/2 cup / 125 mL **white sugar**
1 **omega-3 egg**
1 tsp / 5 mL **vanilla**
11/2 cups / 375 mL **whole-wheat flour**
1/2 tsp / 2 mL **baking soda**
1/4 cup / 50 mL **mini chocolate chips or M&M's baking bits**

1 Preheat oven to 375°F/190°C. Line a cookie sheet with parchment paper.

2 In a medium bowl cream the margarine. Beat in the brown sugar and then the white sugar.

3 Beat in the egg and the vanilla.

4 Stir in the whole-wheat flour, baking soda and chocolate chips.

5 Drop by rounded teaspoonful onto the cookie sheet. Bake for 10 to 12 minutes. Let cool slightly before removing them from the pan.

6 When completely cool store in an airtight container.

Makes 40

WHY MINI CHOCOLATE CHIPS OR M&M'S BAKING BITS?

I really like using the mini chocolate chips or baking bits instead of the regular sized ones. I find they go farther in the recipe. You just feel like you are eating more chocolate per bite! If you only have regular, don't worry, you can use them, but buy a package of mini chocolate chips or baking bits the next time you're out shopping.

TOO SWEET?

Eliminate 1/4 cup / 50 mL of the white sugar.

ONE COOKIE	68 Calories
	0.9 g protein
	3.0 g fat
	0.6 g fiber
	33 mg sodium
	9 g carbohydrate
UHEP	3/4 Fat

Oatmeal Raisin Cookies

Totally Kid-Approved

ROLLED OATS

When you are wandering down the cereal aisle looking for oats, make sure that you are buying the right kind for your recipe. Oats come in many different forms. There are Instant, Quick-Cooking and Rolled Oats. The Rolled Oats are sometimes called Old-Fashioned Oats or Large Flake Oats! If that isn't confusing enough there are also different varieties such as Irish Oats and Scotch Oats that you may come across in the same aisle. So don't just grab the first package you see. For these cookies you need to buy the Old-Fashioned type. Just read the label and buy the right one!

TOO SWEET?

Eliminate 1/4 cup / 50 mL of the white sugar.

These cookies are full of whole grains and raisins. They're lower in fat than most store bought cookies and are made with a healthier fat, canola oil nonhydrogenated margarine.

Here's a little tip when you start to put them onto the cookie sheet—they will spread out while they're baking, so if you are going to get the 48 cookies out of the recipe it's important that you only use a teaspoon of the dough per each cookie.

1/2 cup / 125 mL **nonhydrogenated margarine**
1/2 cup / 125 mL **brown sugar**
1/2 cup / 125 mL **white sugar**
1 **omega-3 egg**
2 tbsp / 25 mL **water**
1/2 tsp / 2 mL **vanilla**
1 1/4 cups / 300 mL **whole-wheat flour**
1 1/4 cups / 300 mL **old-fashioned rolled oats**
1/2 tsp / 2 mL **baking soda**
3/4 cup / 175 mL **raisins**

1 Preheat your oven to 375ºF/190ºC. Line a cookie sheet with parchment paper.

2 In a medium bowl cream the margarine. Beat in the brown sugar and the white sugar. Add the egg, water and vanilla. Beat until light and fluffy.

3 Add the whole-wheat flour, rolled oats and baking soda. Mix until combined.

4 Stir in the raisins.

5 Drop by teaspoonfuls onto the cookie sheet. This will make 48 cookies, if you only use a teaspoonful of batter.

6 Bake for 8 to 10 minutes. Let cool slightly on the cookie sheet, then remove from the pan and let them finish cooling on a wire rack, if you can wait that long. Store in an airtight container.

Makes 4 dozen

ONE COOKIE	
	65 Calories
	1.1 g protein
	2.3 g fat
	0.9 g fiber
	28 mg sodium
	10 g carbohydrate
UHEP	1/2 Fat

Gorp

I have been eating gorp since the late '60s. It was a real "hippie" food back then. A mixture of nuts and dried fruit, it became a fairly popular homemade snack. Somewhere in the '80s, when fitness was first making its mark, the name changed to trail mix. Whatever you call it, it's good! I have added chocolate to make it even better.

2 tbsp / 25 mL **raisins**
2 tbsp / 25 mL **dried, chopped (about 4) apricots**
1/4 cup / 50 mL **almonds or peanuts**
1 tbsp / 15 mL **mini chocolate chips or M&M's baking bits**

1   Mix everything together in a bowl and then divide in half. Put into 2 separate mini plastic bags so you don't eat the whole thing in one sitting! A great snack for the ride home from work.

Makes 2 servings

CHOPPING DRIED APRICOTS
It's a sticky mess at the best of times. Use kitchen scissors! They make the work go fast and it's a great job for your helpers to do! "Hey, let's snip apricots!" Boy, do I know how to entertain kids or what?

ONE SERVING	170 Calories
	3.4 g protein
	8.0 g fat
	3.8 g fiber
	10 mg sodium
	20 g carbohydrate
UHEP	1/2 Vegetables & Fruit
	1/2 Nuts

Super Snackers

Totally Kid-Approved

MICROWAVE METHOD
Put the margarine and the marshmallows into a large microwaveable bowl. Heat on medium-high heat for 2 minutes. Remove from the microwave and stir till melted. Add all the rest of the ingredients, except the chocolate chips. Stir to combine and then add the chocolate chips. Follow the rest of the recipe with step #4.

PEANUT AWARENESS
Lots of schools are now peanut-free zones. My son's school is and that's why we only eat these after school. I never pack them in his lunch. If you or your child has an allergy to nuts, substitute 1/2 cup/125 mL of raisins for the peanuts and an extra 1/2 cup/125 mL of chopped dried apricots for the almonds.

DRIED APRICOTS VS DRIED CRANBERRIES
The research says that dried apricots are very rich in beta-carotene, but I still like dried cranberries better! So if you're like me you may substitute half of the dried apricots with dried cranberries. Liz said it was okay!

Super snackers are a great after-school or after-work treat. Each bar is packed with dried apricots, whole-grain cereal, almonds and don't forget the chocolate chips!

2 tbsp / 25 mL **nonhydrogenated margarine**
40 **large marshmallows**
4 cups / 1 L **whole-grain bran flakes**
2/3 cup / 150 mL **All-Bran Buds**
1/2 cup / 125 mL **almonds—chopped**
1/2 cup / 125 mL **peanuts**
1/2 cup / 125 mL **dried apricots—chopped well**
1/4 cup / 50 mL **mini chocolate chips or M&M's baking bits**

1   In a large pot melt the margarine and the marshmallows over low heat. Stir till melted. Remove from heat.

2   Add the bran flakes, All-Bran Buds, almonds, peanuts and dried apricots. Stir till combined.

3   Quickly stir in the chocolate chips or baking bits; you don't want them to melt.

4   Spoon into a lightly greased 8 x 8-in/20 x 20-cm pan. Dampen hands and press the mixture into the pan. Let cool completely before cutting them. If you are in a hurry, pop them into the fridge for 30 minutes then cut into 16 bars. Store at room temperature, covered.

Makes 16 bars

ONE BAR	204 Calories
	3.4 g protein
	6.0 g fat
	3.8 g fiber
	112 mg sodium
	34 g carbohydrate
UHEP	1/4 Fat
	1/4 Grains
	1/4 Nuts

Date and Nut Loaf

Dates come in several different forms. You can buy them pressed together in a rectangular cake shape or loose in a plastic container. For some reason apparently only the "grocery people" know, the loose ones are found in the fruit and veggie section and the pressed ones are in the baking aisle! It can be very confusing, but, armed with this book, you will be able to circumnavigate most grocery stores instead of wandering around looking for someone who knows something, which, depending on what store you are in, could take days!

1 1/2 cups / 375 mL **water**
2 cups / 500 mL **chopped dates or 1 13-oz / 375-g package pitted dates—chopped**
1 1/2 cups / 375 **mL whole-wheat flour**
1/2 cup / 125 mL **bran**
1/4 cup / 50 mL **walnuts—chopped**
2 tsp / 10 mL **cinnamon**
1 tbsp / 15 mL **baking powder**
1 tsp / 5 mL **baking soda**
1 **omega-3 egg**
1/4 cup / 50 mL **canola oil**
1 cup / 250 mL **brown sugar**

1   Preheat the oven to 350°F/175°C. Lightly grease a loaf pan.

2   In a medium saucepan mix together the water and the chopped dates. Bring to a boil, then reduce heat to simmer. Stir till they form a light paste or, if you have a hand-held blender, here is another wonderful opportunity to use it. Purée the mixture. If you don't have a hand-held blender please turn to page 154 and find out why you really need one.

3   Remove puréed mixture from heat and let cool.

4   In a large bowl mix together the whole-wheat flour, bran, walnuts, cinnamon, baking powder and baking soda.

5   In a medium bowl beat together the egg and oil. Stir in the sugar and cooled date mixture.

6   Add this to the whole-wheat flour mixture. Stir until just combined.

7   Pour into the pan and bake for 45 to 55 minutes or until done.

8   Cool in the pan on a wire rack for 10 minutes. Remove from the pan and continue cooling on the rack.

9   When completely cooled wrap well to store. Tastes great for up to 4 days, if it lasts that long.

Serves 24

ONE SERVING	144 Calories
	2.1 g protein
	3.6 g fat
	2.9 g fiber
	102 mg sodium
	26 g carbohydrate
UHEP	1 Fat
	1/4 Vegetables & Fruit

Date Squares

I was raised on power foods! I just didn't know it! My mom always made us date squares when we were kids. They were loaded with dates, butter and sugar! This updated version isn't quite what Mom made—it's better!

1 13-oz / 375-g pkg. **pitted dates or 2 cups/500 mL**
1 cup / 250 mL **water**
1/4 cup / 50 mL **juice and finely chopped zest of** 1 **orange**
1 1/2 cups / 375 mL **whole-wheat flour**
1 1/2 cups / 375 mL **quick oats**
3/4 cup / 175 mL **brown sugar**
2 tsp / 10 mL **cinnamon**
1/3 cup / 75 mL **canola oil**
1/2 cup / 125 mL **orange juice concentrate** (see page 165)

1 In a medium saucepan, bring the dates and the water to the boil. Reduce heat to low and stir till it becomes a thick paste. Remove from the heat.

2 Stir in the zest and the juice from the orange. Set aside to cool.

3 Preheat the oven to 350°F/175°C. Line a 8 x 8-in/20 x 20-cm pan with foil or parchment paper.

4 In a medium bowl mix together the whole-wheat flour, quick oats, brown sugar and cinnamon.

5 In a small bowl mix together the oil and orange juice concentrate. Pour into the flour mixture. Mix together until the flour mixture looks wet. Pat half of this into the bottom of the pan.

6 Spread the date mixture on top. Spoon over the rest of the flour mixture. Lightly press down.

7 Bake for 30 minutes. Cool completely before cutting it into 16 pieces.

Makes 16

ONE SQUARE	244 Calories
	3.8 g protein
	5.5 g fat
	4.3 g fiber
	5 mg sodium
	45 g carbohydrate
UHEP	1 Fat
	1/2 Vegetables & Fruit
	1/2 Grains

Chocolate Fondue

This is a treat! Albeit a small treat, but there is enough melted chocolate to make you say, "Yum!"

2 oz / 50 g **dark chocolate**
1 tbsp / 15 mL **water**
fruit for dipping

1 Break the chocolate up into pieces. Put it and the water into a small microwaveable bowl. Heat on medium for 30 seconds. Stir. Repeat till almost melted. Stir till fully melted.

2 Dip your fruit in. My choice for dipping is 2 cups/500 mL of strawberries for four servings.

Serves 4

ONE SERVING	79 Calories
	1.2 g protein
	5.1 g fat
	0.8 g fiber
	1 mg sodium
	7 g carbohydrate

Don't Forget to Leave Room for Chocolate Cake!

Totally Kid-Approved

Here it is! A chocolate cake to eat without any guilt (okay maybe a little). Made with whole-wheat flour, canola oil, and chocolate soy milk, it actually tastes like a "real" chocolate cake! Let this become your official birthday/celebration cake. You just keep throwing everything into one bowl and if *that* wasn't good enough—it actually tastes better the next day. The perfect cake for entertaining, it's also an easy make-ahead dessert. It even freezes well! Somebody pinch me!

Serve this with sliced strawberries or raspberries and get in an extra fruit serving as well!

1 cup / 250 mL **whole-wheat flour**
2/3 cup / 150 mL **all purpose flour**
1 1/2 cups / 375 mL **white sugar**
2/3 cup / 150 mL **cocoa powder**
1 1/2 tsp / 7 mL **baking soda**
1/4 cup / 50 mL **canola oil**
1 cup / 250 mL **chocolate soy milk**
2 tsp / 10 mL **lemon juice**
1 **omega-3 egg**
1 4.5 oz / 128 mL jar **strained prunes—no added sugar or starch** (see page 254)
1 tbsp / 15 mL **pure vanilla**

Icing
2 tbsp / 25 mL **nonhydrogenated margarine**
1 oz / 30 g **unsweetened chocolate**
6 tbsp / 90 mL **chocolate soy milk**
2 1/2 cups / 625 mL **icing sugar**
1/3 cup / 75 mL **cocoa powder**

WHICH SOY MILK DO I CHOOSE?

Because all soy milk recipes are different, all soy milks taste different. My two all-time favorite brands are So Good Original and So Nice Original, which is organic as well. My son likes Edensoy Original, but will only drink So Good Chocolate! Experiment. It's up to your own taste buds. For this particular recipe I used So Good Chocolate Soy Milk.

FREEZING TIP

Freeze the cake as is. The next day wrap it in plastic wrap, then put it into a plastic bag, seal it, then pop it back into the freezer. It will stay fresh for 1 month. When you want to serve it, take it out of the freezer the day before the event. Unwrap it and let it sit on the counter until serving time. Another handy tip to make your life easier!

ONE SERVING	
9 x 13-in/ 23 x 33-cm cake with icing, serves 30	151 Calories
	2.2 g protein
	4.0 g fat
	0.7 g fiber
	78 mg sodium
	29 g carbohydrate
UHEP	1 Fat

KID-FRIENDLY TIP

These make great cupcakes. The recipe makes 24 that take 20 to 25 minutes to bake. Ice with the icing recipe and sprinkle with M&M's baking bits for an added kid-appeal. Or bake it in a 9 x 13"/23 x 33 cm pan for 40 minutes. Cool it in the pan and then ice it. A chocolate cake for a weeknight supper or to take to somebody's house.

TO ICE OR NOT TO ICE?

Leave off the icing, bake it in a 9 x 13"/23 x 33 cm pan, let it cool in the pan, sprinkle with icing sugar and cut it into 30 pieces. Still serve it with 1/2 cup/125 mL strawberries or raspberries.

ONE CUPCAKE with icing	189 Calories
	2.8 g protein
	5.0 g fat
	0.9 g fiber
	98 mg sodium
	36 g carbohydrate
UHEP	1 1/4 Fat
ONE SERVING 9 x 13-in / 22 x 33-cm cake without icing sugar, serves 30	95 Calories
	1.8 g protein
	2.5 g fat
	0.6 g fiber
	71 mg sodium
	18 g carbohydrate
UHEP	3/4 Fat

1 Preheat the oven to 350°F/175°C.

2 Lightly spray a 9 x 13-in/23 x 33-cm pan, or line with parchment paper.

3 In a large bowl mix together the whole-wheat flour, all purpose flour, white sugar, cocoa powder and baking soda.

4 Start adding the oil, chocolate soy milk, lemon juice, egg, strained prunes and pure vanilla.

5 Using a hand-mixer or wire whisk beat the ingredients together for 1 minute, scraping the bowl often.

6 Turn the speed up to medium or whisk like your life depended on it and mix for 2 minutes. Pour into prepared pan and bake for 30 to 35 minutes or until a toothpick comes out clean.

7 Cool on a wire rack for 10 minutes then remove from the pan and continue cooling.

8 Prepare icing. Put the margarine, unsweetened chocolate and chocolate soy milk in a microwaveable dish. Heat on medium-low for 1 minute. Stir. Repeat till almost melted. Stir till totally melted. The key is to underdo it! Scorched chocolate is ruined chocolate! And in some countries it's considered a sin.

9 Pour the melted chocolate into a medium bowl. Don't lick this—it hasn't any sugar in it yet! Add the icing sugar and the cocoa powder and beat till smooth. If it is too thick add a little bit of chocolate soy milk until you reach the desired thickness. Lick beaters if desired.

10 Ice cooled cake. Lick bowl. The cake can now be eaten immediately or the next day. Remember that tomorrow it will taste better! Your choice.

Serves 30

Pantry and Equipment List

Once you buy this book you will need certain foods in your house as staples. The old saying, "You are only as good a cook as your pantry is stocked!" is totally true.

Some of these ingredients are very common, like vinegar and extra virgin olive oil, which you probably have kicking around your kitchen already. Some ingredients like long-grain brown rice and silken tofu, you may not.

Read the recipes through, do a pantry inventory, and write down the things that you'll need. Don't throw all your old stuff out; it's expensive, and you can replace the old foods with the new ones as you go along.

There are some "different" ingredients that you may think aren't worth adding to a recipe, like chili garlic sauce. Trust me, I only included items that made a flavor impact and that were easy to find in most grocery stores. Happy shopping and cooking.

PANTRY AND EQUIPMENT LIST

BAKING INGREDIENTS

Baking powder
Baking soda
Bran (wheat and oat)
Brown sugar
Cocoa powder
Cornmeal
Cornstarch
Currants
Dark chocolate
Dried fruit—
    Apricots
    Cranberries
    Dates
    Prunes
    Raisins
Flaxseed
Honey
Icing sugar
M&M's baking bits
Maple syrup
Mini chocolate chips
Molasses
Pumpkin purée
Pure vanilla extract
Raisins
Rolled oats—old-fashioned
    and quick-cooking
Strained prunes—4.5-oz
    /128-mL jar
Wheat germ
Whole-wheat flour

OTHER INGREDIENTS

Apple cider vinegar
Balsamic vinegar
Beano
Bulgur
Canned apricots
Canned beans in tomato
    sauce
Canned black beans
Canned or tetra pak package
    of chicken stock—low
    sodium where available
Canned kidney beans
Canned lentils
Canned plum tomatoes
Canned salmon
Canned tomato paste
Canned vegetable stock—
    low sodium where
    available
Canned water-packed
    tuna—low sodium
Cereal—All Bran Buds
Couscous
Evaporated milk—fat free
    and 2%
Fresh ginger
lower-sodium soy sauce

Nuts—
    Almonds
    Cashews
    Peanuts
    Walnuts
Oils—canola and extra
    virgin olive
Peanut butter—chunky or
    smooth
Quinoa
Red wine vinegar
Rice vinegar
Rice
    Long-grain brown rice
    Short-grain brown rice
    Wild rice
Split peas
White vinegar
Whole-wheat pasta—
    Lasagne
    Penne
    Rotini
    Spaghetti
Worcestershire sauce

REFRIGERATED INGREDIENTS

Cheese—light—your choice
Curry paste
Dijon mustard—grainy and
    regular
Eggs—omega-3
Fruits—your choice
Hot pepper jelly
Hot peppers
Ketchup
Low-fat mayonnaise
Mango chutney
Marmalade
Milk—skim and buttermilk
Mustard—horseradish and
    regular
Nonhydrogenated margarine
Olives—black and green
Oyster sauce
Salsa
Silken tofu
Soy beverage—your choice
Sundried tomatoes packed
    in olive oil
Vegetables—your choice
Yogurt—low fat and
    French Vanilla

HERBS AND SPICES

Allspice
Basil
Black pepper
Cayenne
Chili powder
Cinnamon
Curry powder
Dried oregano
Dried tarragon
Dried thyme
Garlic
Ground cinnamon
Ground cloves
Ground coriander
Ground cumin
Nutmeg
Onion powder
Paprika
Red pepper flakes
Salt
Turmeric
White pepper

FROZEN INGREDIENTS

Banana chunks
Blueberries
Corn
Cranberries
Frozen concentrated
    orange juice
Frozen concentrated
    raspberry cocktail
Green beans
Peas
Raspberries
Strawberries
Whole-wheat tortillas

EQUIPMENT

Food processor or free-
    standing blender
Garlic press
Hand-held blender
Lemon juicer
Parchment paper
Resealable plastic bags
Salad spinner
Zester

APPENDIX

How healthy are you? Use these guidelines to see how well your health rates. If you haven't had your blood pressure or blood cholesterol checked lately, do so the next time you visit your family doctor.

Healthy Blood Cholesterol Levels

LDL cholesterol
Less than 100 mg/dL (2.6 mmol/L)

Total cholesterol
Less than 200 mg/dL (5.2 mmol/L)

HDL cholesterol
Greater than 45 mg/dL (1.17 mmol/L) is acceptable; equal to or greater than 60 mg/dL is optimal (1.56 mmol/L)

Triglyceride Levels
Less than 150 mg/dL (2.3 mmol/L) is healthy.
Over 400 mg/dL (4.5 mmol/L) is high.

Healthy Blood Pressure
Less than 120/80 mmHg is optimal.
High blood pressure is greater than or equal to 140/90 mmHg.

Waist Circumference
If you carry excess weight in your abdominal area you are at higher risk for the development of disease including diabetes and heart disease.

High risk for men is a waist greater than 40 inches (102 cm) around.

High risk for women is a waist greater than 35 inches (88 cm) around.

Future Possibilities
In the future your doctor may also measure or monitor others factors in your blood, including homocysteine, c-reactive protein and lipoprotein (a). Each of these measures appears to help determine the risk of heart disease.

Healthy Weight Guidelines

Early diagnosis of an unhealthy weight (also referred to as body mass index) can potentially aid in the prevention of disease and provide advance warning of any health problems.

HEIGHT	HEALTHY WEIGHT	CAUTION ZONE	HEALTH RISK ZONE
4'11" (150 cm)	99–123 pounds	124–133 pounds	over 133 pounds
5' (153 cm)	102–127 pounds	128–138 pounds	over 138 pounds
5'1" (155 cm)	106–131 pounds	132–143 pounds	over 143 pounds
5'2" (158 cm)	109–135 pounds	136–147 pounds	over 147 pounds
5'3" (160 cm)	113–140 pounds	141–152 pounds	over 152 pounds
5'4" (163 cm)	116–144 pounds	145–157 pounds	over 157 pounds
5'5" (165 cm)	120–149 pounds	150–162 pounds	over 162 pounds
5'6" (168 cm)	124–154 pounds	155–167 pounds	over 167 pounds
5'7" (170 cm)	127–158 pounds	159–172 pounds	over 172 pounds
5'8" (173 cm)	131–163 pounds	164–177 pounds	over 177 pounds
5'9" (175 cm)	135–168 pounds	169–182 pounds	over 182 pounds
5'10" (178 cm)	139–173 pounds	174–188 pounds	over 188 pounds
5'11" (180 cm)	143–178 pounds	179–193 pounds	over 193 pounds
6' (183 cm)	147–183 pounds	184–199 pounds	over 199 pounds
6'1" (185 cm)	151–188 pounds	189–204 pounds	over 204 pounds
6'2" (188 cm)	155–193 pounds	194–210 pounds	over 210 pounds
6'3" (190 cm)	160–199 pounds	200–216 pounds	over 216 pounds

Please note

To convert pounds to kilograms divide by 2.2.

This chart should not be used to evaluate the weight of children, the frail elderly, serious body-builders, or pregnant or breast-feeding women. If your extra weight comes from muscle, not fat, you may have a high body mass index even though you are healthy.

NUTRITION ANALYSIS SUMMARY CHART

Note: Where sodium values may differ according to stock used, the first listed value is presented here.

RECIPES	Servings	Calories	Protein	Fat	Fiber	Sodium	Carbo-hydrates
SALADS							
House Dressing	4	58	0.2	4.9	0.1	5.1	4
Unbelievably Delicious Raspberry Salad Dressing	4	55	0.2	4.6	0.1	0.5	3
Tarragon Vinaigrette	4	58	0.1	4.7	0.2	0.3	5
Mango Chutney Dressing	4	78	0.1	4.7	0.2	147	10
Strawberry and Spinach Salad							
without almonds	4	145	2.2	9.8	3.4	57	15
with almonds	4	214	4.7	15.8	4.8	57	17
Romaine with Feta and Blueberries	4	145	3.7	7.2	2.7	19	19
Spinach Salad	4	213	6.9	13.1	5.6	55	20
Carrot Salad	6	101	1.9	4.4	2.5	86	15
Grape Tomato Salad	4	68	0.9	5.7	1.3	65	5
without olives	4	60	0.9	5	1.1	8	4
SOUPS							
Broccoli Soup	6	66	4.8	0.4	2.4	410	12
Marvelous Minestrone	6	244	9.8	4.4	12.1	722	38
Quick and Hearty Chicken Noodle Soup	4	293	37.2	4.4	3.4	1068	25
Lentil Soup	6	128	7.3	0.5	4.4	412	25
Black Bean Soup	4	173	10	1	10.1	473	33
with yogurt and cilantro	4	192	11.5	1.4	10.1	496	35
Skinny Squash Soup	6	125	3.7	3.6	3.7	581	23
Gazpacho	8	60	2.1	1.8	2.4	167	11
VEGGIES							
Honey Glazed Carrots	4	67	0.6	3	1.8	39	10
Honey Dijon Glazed Carrots	4	68	0.6	3	1.8	39	10
Tomatoes with Fresh Basil	4	33	0.6	2.5	0.7	4	3
Quickie Sweet Potatoes	4	94	1.5	0.2	1.4	10	22
Acorn Squash with Maple Syrup	4	66	1.6	2.2	1.6	17	12
Butternut Squash with Brown Sugar and Cinnamon	6	73	2.2	1.7	2.5	15	15
Sweet Spaghetti Squash	4	43	0.8	2.1	0.8	15	6
Grilled Veggie Salad	4	86	2.5	3.9	2.6	30	13
Yellow and Red Peppers with Vidalia Onions	6	68	1.4	3.4	1.9	3	10
Honey Lime Sweet Potatoes	4	134	1.3	2.6	1.4	10	27
Sweet Potato Coins	4	128	1.6	5.3	1.7	11	20
Asparagus with Balsamic Vinegar	4	58	4.2	2.4	2.1	126	8
Broccoli, Red Pepper and Fresh Ginger	4	61	2.5	3.8	3.5	20	6
Stir-Fried Broccoli with Cashews	4	157	5.6	10.9	3	287	12

RECIPES	Servings	Calories	Protein	Fat	Fiber	Sodium	Carbo-hydrates
Stir-Fried Brussels Sprouts and Carrots	4	76	2.1	4.6	2.8	84	8
Brussels Sprouts with Maple Syrup	4	59	1.5	3.2	1.7	31	7
Roasted Garlic Potatoes	4	147	2.9	4.8	2.1	8	25
GRAINS							
Wild and Brown Rice	6	113	3.4	0.8	1.2	326	23
Brown Rice with Dried Cranberries and Orange	6	130	3.3	1	1.8	327	27
Short-Grain Brown Rice Risotto with Kale and Squash	6	203	7.5	2.8	4.9	587	39
Bulgar Pilaf	6	123	4.3	3.6	4.7	330	20
Orange Bulgar	6	100	3.2	0.3	4.3	5	22
Spicy Bulgar Pilaf	6	132	4.2	3.6	5.4	335	23
Quinoa Pilaf	8	113	3.1	3.7	1.7	182	18
Barley Risotto	8	113	3.9	3.5	0.6	364	17
PASTA							
Asian Noodle Salad	4	350	14.4	14.5	9	516	46
Rotini with Plum Tomatoes and Lentils	4	356	17.2	7.5	10.6	802	57
Pasta Primavera	4	248	10.6	5.8	6.9	329	41
Rotini with Feta and Tomatoes	4	276	6	8	4.4	93	35
Mairlyn's Amazing Tomato Sauce	8	106	2.8	4.2	5.2	440	15
with 1 1/2 cups (375 mL) pasta	8	425	13.8	6.2	10.2	442	79
Spinach Lasagna							
with Mairlyn's Amazing Tomato Sauce	6	433	25.5	16	10.3	699	47
Tuna Pasta Salad	4	307	23.2	6.7	5.9	210	42
Spicy Turkey Pasta Sauce	8	176	9.5	5	6.4	815	23
with 1 cup (250 mL) cooked whole-wheat spaghetti	8	389	16.8	6.3	9.8	816	66
POULTRY							
Chicken with Mango and Apricots	4	331	32.3	3.7	0.6	547	40
Chicken Biriyani	4	416	37.7	9.2	1.9	594	44
Chicken Tarragon	4	234	34.3	5.2	0.6	564	6
Sundried Tomato Pesto with Chicken and Rotini	4	442	42.5	9.5	2.9	251	46
Ginger Chicken Stir-Fry	4	385	37.1	7	6.3	741	46
Chicken with Dried Cranberries	4	283	31.3	3.7	0.9	83	30
Chicken Mango Salad	2	281	18.5	13.9	4.3	70	21
Lemon Chicken	4	198	31.3	3.6	0.3	76	9
Raspberry Chicken	4	197	31.1	3.6	0.1	75	9

Note: Where sodium values may differ according to stock used, the first listed value is presented here.

RECIPES	Servings	Calories	Protein	Fat	Fiber	Sodium	Carbo-hydrates
Chicken Burgers							
on a hamburger bun	6	271	22.1	10.4	3	378	30
not on a hamburger bun	6	158	17.9	7.8	1.3	182	11
Salsa Baked Chicken	4	227	32.5	3.6	0.3	74	10
SEAFOOD							
Wasabi Salmon	4	186	18.6	10	0.1	196	4
Spicy Salmon Cakes	7	214	13	10.6	2.4	426	16
with Dippy Sauce	7	237	13	12.8	2.4	426	17
with Citrus Sauce	7	226	13.2	10.6	2.5	474	19
Baked Salmon with Fresh Citrus	4	218	18.7	10.1	0.5	56	18
Company's Comin' Salmon	4	182	18.5	10	0	55	2
Baked Salmon with Fresh Ginger	4	255	19.6	10.1	0.4	691	19
Salmon with Mango Salsa	4	201	18.5	10	0.7	56	8
Poached Salmon with Mairlyn's World Famous Lime Mayo	4	204	18.4	13.3	0	54	1
Salmon Teriyaki	4	191	18.9	10	0	476	5
"Really Great Salmon!"	4	180	19	10	0.1	486	2
Creamy Dilled Salmon	4	186	19	10.2	0.	70	3
Sunset Shrimp	4	300	23	6	3	147	34
Salmon Chowder	4	333	28	10.4	4.5	890	33
BEEF							
Beef and Broccoli Stir-Fry	4	275	33.8	10.7	3.4	455	12
Beef Kebobs	4	273	33.4	6.9	3.7	96	20
BEANS							
Summer Fiesta Chickpea Salad	4	258	8.5	6.7	8.5	221	43
Hummus with Roasted Red Peppers	8	117	4.5	3	3.8	102	19
Mairlyn's World Famous Beans and Rice	8	275	11.4	4.1	12.9	562	49
Remarkable Refried Beans	4	157	9.3	2.1	9.4	136	27
Burritos	4	337	17.8	6.4	14.4	655	53
Nachos	2	256	12.7	65.4	9.3	412	40
Amazing Black Bean Quesadillas	4	452	22.7	11.1	13.1	589	64
Jerk Black Beans	4	167	8.8	4.1	9.1	116	25
South of the Border Lasagna	4	406	27.4	9.6	12.2	484	59
Out-of-this-World Chili	8	248	15.8	5	13	608	36
Mexican Lentil Casserole	6	281	15.7	8.7	7.6	780	37
Taco-Taco Salad							
with tortillas	4	369	22.6	11.3	12.5	500	49
without tortillas	4	274	19.9	9.3	10.8	358	34
Jazzy Beans	4	209	7.7	5.5	7.1	502	33
So Soya+ Stir-Fry	4	141	12.4	5.1	6.6	578	16

RECIPES	Servings	Calories	Protein	Fat	Fiber	Sodium	Carbo-hydrates
FRUIT							
Super Chocolate Banana Soy Shake	1	227	7.5	3.6	2.8	141	45
Super Chocolate Banana Tofu Milkshake	1	315	11.5	4.6	3.5	29	60
Super Berry Shake	1	257	10.6	3.7	2.3	3	49
Super Soy Strawberry Smoothie	1	187	9.3	5	1.8	158	26
Big Blue Berry Purple Smoothie	1	233	9.2	5.4	2.9	141	40
Strawberries with French Vanilla Yogurt	1	115	6.6	1.3	2.4	81	30
Dried Fruit Compote	4	216	2.1	0.4	4.4	18	54
Frozen Raspberry Yogurt	4	106	4.1	0.8	1.3	40	21
Blueberry Nectarine Crisp	8	244	3.2	8	4.2	8	44
MUFFINS, PANCAKES AND FRENCH TOAST							
Banana Chocolate Chip Muffins	12	190	5.2	5.8	6	217	31
Super Nutritious Chocolate Chip Bran Muffins	12	234	6.2	6	7.7	169	41
Pumpkin Chocolate Chip Muffins	12	210	6.3	6	8	250	36
Blueberry Muffins	12	201	4.8	6.3	4.5	211	32
Cranberry Orange Muffins	12	230	6.17	6.5	6.7	188	41
Apple and Oat Pancakes	4	339	15.1	7.5	9.4	474	58
with apple sauce	4	395	15.3	7.8	11.7	486	72
Whole-Wheat Blueberry Buttermilk Pancakes	4	303	14	8.9	7.8	505	44
French Toast	4	226	12.2	8.9	5.6	210	27
COOKIES, LOAVES, TREATS AND CAKE							
Chocolate Chip Cookies	40	68	0.9	3	0.6	33	9
Oatmeal Raisin Cookies	48	65	1.1	2.3	0.9	28	10
Gorp	2	170	3.4	8	3.8	10	20
Super Snackers	16	204	3.4	6	3.8	112	34
Date and Nut Loaf	24	144	2.1	3.6	2.9	102	26
Date Squares	16	244	3.8	5.5	4.3	5	45
Chocolate Fondue	4	79	1.2	5.1	0.8	1	7
Don't Forget to Leave Room for Chocolate Cake!	30	151	2.2	4	0.7	78	29
cupcakes	24	189	2.8	5	0.9	98	36
without icing	30	95	1.8	2.5	0.6	71	18

UHEP SUMMARY CHART

RECIPES	Servings	Beans	Eggs	Fat	Fish
SALADS					
House Dressing	4			1	
Unbelievably Delicious Raspberry	4			1	
** Salad Dressing**					
Tarragon Vinaigrette	4			1	
Mango Chutney Dressing	4			1	
Strawberry and Spinach Salad					
** without almonds**	4			2	
** with almonds**	4			2	
Romaine with Feta and Blueberries	4			1	
Spinach Salad	4			1/2	
Carrot Salad	6				
Grape Tomato Salad	4			1	
** without olives**	4			1	
SOUPS					
Broccoli Soup	6				
Marvelous Minestrone	6	3/4		3/4	
Quick and Hearty Chicken Noodle Soup	4				
Lentil Soup	6	3/4			
Black Bean Soup	4	1			
** with yogurt and cilantro**	4	1			
Skinny Squash Soup	6			3/4	
Gazpacho	8			1/4	
VEGGIES					
Honey Glazed Carrots	4			3/4	
Honey Dijon Glazed Carrots	4			3/4	
Tomatoes with Fresh Basil	4			1/2	
Quickie Sweet Potatoes	4				
Acorn Squash with Maple Syrup	4			1/2	
Butternut Squash with Brown Sugar	6			1/2	
** and Cinnamon**					
Sweet Spaghetti Squash	4			1/2	
Grilled Veggie Salad	4			3/4	
Yellow and Red Peppers with	6			3/4	
** Vidalia Onions**					
Honey Lime Sweet Potatoes	4			1/2	
Sweet Potato Coins	4			1	
Asparagus with Balsamic Vinegar	4			1/2	
Broccoli, Red Pepper and Fresh Ginger	4			3/4	
Stir-Fried Broccoli with Cashews	4			1/2	

Flax	Vegetables and Fruit	Grains	Meat	Milk	Nuts	Soy
	3					
	3				1/2	
	2			1/4		
	2 1/2				1/2	
	1 1/2					
	1					
	1					
	1 1/4					
	2 1/2	1/4				
	1 3/4	1	1			
	1					
	1/2					
	1/2					
	1 1/2					
	1					
	1					
	1					
	1					
	1					
	1					
	1					
	1					
	1 1/2					
	1					
	1					
	1					
	1					
	2 1/4					
	2 1/4				1/2	

RECIPES	Servings	Beans	Eggs	Fat	Fish
Stir-Fried Brussels Sprouts and Carrots	4			1	
Brussels Sprouts with Maple Syrup	4			3/4	
Roasted Garlic Potatoes	4			1	
GRAINS					
Wild and Brown Rice	6				
Brown Rice with Dried Cranberries and Orange	6				
Short-Grain Brown Rice Risotto with Kale and Squash	6				
Bulgar Pilaf	6			3/4	
Orange Bulgar	6				
Spicy Bulgar Pilaf	6			3/4	
Quinoa Pilaf	8				
Barley Risotto	8			1/2	
PASTA					
Asian Noodle Salad	4				
Rotini with Plum Tomatoes and Lentils	4	1		1	
Pasta Primavera	4			1/2	
Rotini with Feta and Tomatoes	4				
Mairlyn's Amazing Tomato Sauce	8			1	
with 11/2 cups (375 mL) pasta	8			1	
Spinach Lasagna					
with Mairlyn's Amazing Tomato Sauce	6			1/2	
Tuna Pasta Salad	4			1	4
Spicy Turkey Pasta Sauce	8			3/4	
with 1 cup (250 mL) cooked whole-wheat spaghetti	8			3/4	
POULTRY					
Chicken with Mango and Apricots	4				
Chicken Biriyani	4			1	
Chicken Tarragon	4				
Sundried Tomato Pesto with Chicken and Rotini	4				
Ginger Chicken Stir-Fry	4			1/2	
Chicken with Dried Cranberries	4				
Chicken Mango Salad	2			1/2	
Lemon Chicken	4				
Raspberry Chicken	4				

Flax	Vegetables and Fruit	Grains	Meat	Milk	Nuts	Soy
	2					
	1					
	2 1/2					
		1				
	1/4	1				
	1 3/4	1				
		1				
	1/4	1				
	1/2	1				
		1				
	1/4	1/2				
	4 3/4	1			1	
	2	1 1/2				
	3	1 1/2		1/4		
	2	1 1/2		1/2		
	1					
	1	3				
	2	2		1		
	1 1/2	1 1/2				
	1		1			
	1	2	1			
	1		1			
		1 1/2	1	1/4		
			1			
	1/4	2	1	1/2		
	3 1/2	1	1			
	1/2		1			
	3		1/2		1/2	
			1			
			1			

RECIPES	Servings	Beans	Eggs	Fat	Fish
Chicken Burgers					
on a hamburger bun	6				
not on a hamburger bun	6				
Salsa Baked Chicken	4				
SEAFOOD					
Wasabi Salmon	4				1
Spicy Salmon Cakes	7			3/4	1
with Dippy Sauce	7			2	1
with Citrus Sauce	7			3/4	1
Baked Salmon with Fresh Citrus	4				1
Company's Comin' Salmon	4				1
Baked Salmon with Fresh Ginger	4				1
Salmon with Mango Salsa	4				1
Poached Salmon with Mairlyn's World Famous Lime Mayo	4			1/2	1
Salmon Teriyaki	4				1
"Really Great Salmon!"	4				1
Creamy Dilled Salmon	4				1
Sunset Shrimp	4			3/4	1
Salmon Chowder	4				1
BEEF					
Beef and Broccoli Stir-Fry	4			1	
Beef Kebobs	4				
BEANS					
Summer Fiesta Chickpea Salad	4	1		1	
Hummus with Roasted Red Peppers	8	1/2		3/4	
Mairlyn's World Famous Beans and Rice	8	1		1/2	
Remarkable Refried Beans	4	1		1/4	
Burritos	4	1		1/4	
Nachos	2	1			
Amazing Black Bean Quesadillas	4	1			
Jerk Black Beans	4	1		3/4	
South of the Border Lasagna	4	1			
Out-of-this-World Chili	8	1		1	
Mexican Lentil Casserole	6	3/4		3/4	
Taco-Taco Salad					
with tortillas	4	1		1	
without tortillas	4	1		1	
Jazzy Beans	4	1		1	

Flax	Vegetables and Fruit	Grains	Meat	Milk	Nuts	Soy
		2¼	1			
		¼	1			
	½		1			
		1				
		1				
		1				
	¼					
	½					
		1½				
	3¼			½		
	2		1			
	2½		1			
	2¾					
	½					
	1½	¾				
	2	1		¼		
	3¼	2		½		
	1	2		½		
	2½	¾		1		
	1					¾
	1½			½		
	1¾	1	½			
	1¾		½			

RECIPES	Servings	Beans	Eggs	Fat	Fish
So Soya+ Stir-Fry	4			1	
FRUIT					
Super Chocolate Banana Soy Shake	1				
Super Chocolate Banana Tofu Milkshake	1				
Super Berry Shake	1				
Super Soy Strawberry Smoothie	1				
Big Blue Berry Purple Smoothie	1				
Strawberries with French Vanilla Yogurt	1				
Dried Fruit Compote	4				
Frozen Raspberry Yogurt	4				
Blueberry Nectarine Crisp	8			1 1/2	
MUFFINS, PANCAKES AND FRENCH TOAST					
Banana Chocolate Chip Muffins	12				
Super Nutritious Chocolate Chip Bran Muffins	12				
Pumpkin Chocolate Chip Muffins	12				
Blueberry Muffins	12		1		
Cranberry Orange Muffins	12				
Apple and Oat Pancakes	4				
with apple sauce	4				
Whole-Wheat Blueberry Buttermilk Pancakes	4			1	
French Toast	4		1		
COOKIES, LOAVES, TREATS AND CAKE					
Chocolate Chip Cookies	40			3/4	
Oatmeal Raisin Cookies	48			1/2	
Gorp	2				
Super Snackers	16			1/4	
Date and Nut Loaf	24			1	
Date Squares	16			1	
Chocolate Fondue	4				
Don't Forget to Leave Room for Chocolate Cake!	30			1	
cupcakes	24			1 1/4	
without icing	30			3/4	

Flax	Vegetables and Fruit	Grains	Meat	Milk	Nuts	Soy
	2¹/₂					1
	2					1
	2			¹/₂		1
	2			¹/₂		1
	1					1
	1					1
	2			¹/₄		
	3					
	1			¹/₄		
	1¹/₂	¹/₄				
1	¹/₂	1¹/₂				
1		1¹/₂				
1		1¹/₂				
	¹/₄	1¹/₂				
1	¹/₄	1				
1	¹/₂	3		¹/₂		
1	1¹/₂	3		¹/₂		
	¹/₂	3		¹/₄		
		2		¹/₄		
	¹/₂				¹/₂	
		¹/₄			¹/₄	
	¹/₄					
	¹/₂	¹/₂				
	1					

BIBLIOGRAPHY

Healthy-For-You Fats

Angerer, P., et al. "n-3 Polyunsaturated Fatty Acids and the Cardiovascular System." *Current Opinion in Lipidology* 11 (2000): 57–63.

Ascherio, A., et al. "Dietary Fat and Risk of Coronary Heart Disease in Men: Cohort Follow-up study in the United States." *British Medical Journal* 313 (1996): 84–90.

Ascherio, A., et al. "Trans Fatty Acids and Coronary Heart Disease." *The New England Journal of Medicine* 340 (1999): 1994–98.

Asher, M., et al. "Intake of Trans Fatty Acids and Prevalence of Childhood Asthma and Allergies in Europe. ISAAC Steering Committee." *Lancet* 353 (1999): 2040–41.

Bartsch, H., et al. "Dietary Polyunsaturated Fatty Acids and Cancers of the Breast and Colorectum: Emerging Evidence for Their Role as Risk Modifiers." *Carcinogenesis* 20 (1999): 2209–18.

Baskou, D. "Olive Oil." *World Review of Nutrition and Diet* 87 (2000): 56–77.

Bruinsma, K. "Dieting, Essential Fatty Acid Intake, and Depression." *Nutrition Reviews* 58 (2000): 98–108.

Callaway, W. "The Role of Fat-Modified Foods in the American Diet." *Nutrition Today* 33 (1998): 156–62.

Colditz, G., et al. "The Nurses' Health Study: 20-Year Contribution to the Understanding of Health Among Women." *Journal of Women's Health* 6 (1997): 49–62.

Connor, W. "Importance of n-3 Fatty Acids in Health and Disease." *American Journal of Clinical Nutrition* 71 (2000): 171S–175S.

Coulston, A. "The Role of Dietary Fats in Plant-Based Diets." *American Journal of Clinical Nutrition* 70 (1999): 512S–515S.

Denke, M., et al. "Individual Cholesterol Variation in Response to a Margarine or Butter Based Diet." *Journal of the American Medical Association* 284 (2000): 2740–47.

Hu, F., et al. "Dietary Intake of Alpha-Linolenic Acid and Risk of Fatal Ischemic Heart Disease Among Women." *American Journal of Clinical Nutrition* 69 (1999): 890–97.

Hu, F., et al. "Types of Dietary Fat and Risk of Coronary Heart Disease: A Critical Review." *Journal of the American College of Nutrition* 20 (2001): 5–19.

Kaklamani, L., et al. "Dietary Factors in Relation to Rheumatoid Arthritis: A Role for Olive Oil and Cooked Vegetables?" *American Journal of Clinical Nutrition* 71 (2000): 1010.

Katan, M. "Trans Fatty Acids and Plasma Lipoproteins." *Nutrition Reviews* 58 (2000): 188–91.

Kris-Etherton, P., et al. "Monounsaturated Fatty Acids and Risk of Cardiovascular Disease." *Circulation* 100 (1999): 1253–57.

Kris-Etherton, P., et al. "Polyunsaturated Fatty Acids in the Food Chain in the United States." *American Journal of Clinical Nutrition* 71 (2000): 179S–188S.

Lichtenstein, A., "Dietary Trans Fatty Acid." *Journal of Cardiopulmonary Rehabilitation* 20 (2000): 143–46.

Lorgeril, M., et al. "Mediterranean Alpha-Linolenic Acid-Rich Diet in Secondary Prevention of Coronary Heart Disease." *Lancet* 343 (1994): 1454–59.

Lorgeril, M., et al. "Mediterranean Diet, Traditional Risk Factors, and the Rate of Cardiovascular Complications After Myocardial Infarction." *Circulation* 99 (1999): 779–85.

Owen, R., et al. "The Antioxidant/Anticancer Potential of Phenolic Compounds Isolated from Olive Oil." *European Journal of Cancer* 36 (2000): 1235–47.

Rose, D., and Connolly, F. "Omega-3 Fatty Acids as Cancer Chemopreventive Agents." *Pharmacology and Therapeutics* 83 (1999): 217–41.

Simopoulos, A. "Essential Fatty Acids in Health and Chronic Disease." *American Journal of Clinical Nutrition* 70 (1999): 560S–595S.

Simopoulos, A., et al. "Essentiality of and Recommended Dietary Intakes for Omega-6 and Omega-3 Fatty Acids." *Annals of Nutrition Metabolism* 43 (1999): 127–30.

Simopoulos, A., et al. "Evolutionary Aspects of Omega-3 Fatty Acids in the Food Supply." *Prostaglandins, Leukotrienes and Essential Fatty Acids* 60 (1999): 421–29.

Stampfer, M., et al. "Primary Prevention of Coronary Heart Disease in Women Through Diet and Lifestyle." *New England Journal of Medicine* 343 (2000): 16–22.

Visioli, F. and Galli, C. "The Effect of Minor Constituents of Olive Oil on Cardiovascular Disease: New Findings." *Nutrition Reviews* 56 (1998): 142–47.

Phenomenal Vegetables and Fruit

Bone, R., et al. "Lutein and Zeaxanthin in the Eyes, Serum and Diet of Human Subjects." *Experimental Eye Research* 71 (2000): 239–45.

Cohen, J., et al. "Fruit and Vegetable Intakes and Prostate Cancer Risk." *Journal of the National Cancer Institute* 92 (2000): 61–68.

Craig, W. "Health-Promoting Properties of Common Herbs." *American Journal of Clinical Nutrition* 70 (1999): 491S–499S.

Feskanich, D., et al. "Prospective Study of Fruit and Vegetable Consumption and Risk of Lung Cancer Among Men and Women." *Journal of the National Cancer Institute* 92 (2000): 1812–23.

Gandini, S., et al. "Meta-Analysis of Studies on Breast Cancer Risk and Diet: The Role of Fruit and Vegetable Consumption and the Intake of Associated Micronutrients." *European Journal of Cancer* 36 (2000): 636–46.

Getahun, S. and Chung, F. "Conversion of Glucosinolates to Isothiocyanates in Humans after Ingestion of Cooked Watercress." *Cancer Epidemiology, Biomarkers & Prevention* 8 (1999): 447–51.

Giovannucci, E. "Tomatoes, Tomato-Based Products, Lycopene and Cancer: Review of the Epidemiologic Literature." *Journal of the National Cancer Institute* 91 (1999): 317–31.

Halliwell, B. "Why and How Should We Measure Oxidative DNA Damage in Nutritional Studies? How Far Have We Come?" *American Journal of Clinical Nutrition* 72 (2000): 1082–87.

Hecht, S. "Inhibition of Carcinogenesis by Isothiocyanates." *Drug Metabolsim Reviews* 32 (2000): 395–411.

Hollman, P., and Katan, M. "Dietary Flavonoids: Intake, Healthy Effects and Bioavailability." *Food and Chemical Toxicology* 37 (1999): 937–42.

Joshipura, K., et al. "Fruit and Vegetable Intake in Relation to Risk of Ischemic Stroke." *Journal of the American Medical Association* 282 (1999): 1233–39.

Keevil, J., et al. "Grape Juice, But not Orange Juice or Grapefruit Juice Inhibits Human Platelet Aggregation." *Journal of Nutrition* 130 (2000): 53–56.

Kurilich, A., et al. "Carotene, Tocopherol, and Ascorbate Contents in Subspecies of Brassica Oleracea." *Journal of Agricultural Food Chemistry* 47 (1999): 1576–81.

Lampe, J. "Health Effects of Vegetables and Fruit: Assessing Mechanisms of Action in Human Experimental Studies." *American Journal of Nutrition* 7 (1999): 475S–490S.

Michaud, D., et al. "Intake of Specific Carotenoids and Risk of Lung Cancer in 2 Prospective US Cohorts." *American Journal of Clinical Nutrition* 72 (2000): 990–97.

Miller, H., et al. "Antioxidant Content of Whole Grain Breakfast Cereals, Fruits and Vegetables." *Journal of the American College of Nutrition* 19 (2000): 312S–319S.

Pietta, P. "Flavonoids as Antioxidants." *Journal of Natural Products* 63 (2000): 1035–42.

Sacks, F., et al. "A Dietary Approach to Prevent Hypertension: A Review of the Dietary Approaches to Stop Hypertension (DASH) Study." *Clinical Cardiology* 22 (1999): 6S–10S.

Sergio, P., and Russell, R. "B-Carotene and Other Carotenoids as Antioxidants." *Journal of the American College of Nutrition* 18 (1999): 426–33.

Thompson, H., et al. "Effect of Increased Vegetable and Fruit Consumption on Markers of Oxidative Cellular Damage." *Carcinogenesis* 20 (1999): 2261–66.

Thurnham, D., and Clewes, C. "Optimal Nutrition: Vitamin A and the Carotenoids." *Proceedings of the Nutrition Society* 58 (1999): 449–57.

Veer, P., et al. "Fruits and Vegetables in the Prevention of Cancer and Cardiovascular Disease." *Public Health Nutrition* 3 (2000): 103–07.

Wonderful Whole Grains

Adams, J., and Engstrom, A. "Helping Consumers Achieve Recommended Intakes of Whole Grains." *Journal of the American College of Nutrition* 19 (2000): 339S–344S.

Anderson, J., et al. "Cholesterol-Lowering Effects of Psyllium Intake Adjunctive to Diet Therapy in Men and Women with Hypercholesterolemia: Meta-Analysis of 8 Controlled Trials." *American Journal of Clinical Nutrition* 71 (2000): 472–79.

Anderson, J., et al. "Whole Grain Foods and Heart Disease Risk." *Journal of the American College of Nutrition* 19 (2000): 291S–299S.

Baublis, A., et al. "Potential of Wheat-Based Breakfast Cereals as a Source of Dietary Antioxidants." *Journal of the American College of Nutrition* 19 (2000): 308S–311S.

Cleveland, L., et al. "Dietary Intake of Whole Grains." *Journal of the American College of Nutrition* 19 (2000): 331S–338S.

Halifrisch, J., and Behall, K. "Mechanisms of the Effects of Grains on Insulin and Glucose Responses." *Journal of the American College of Nutrition* 19 (2000): 320S–325S.

Jacobs, D., et al. "Is Whole Grain Intake Associated with Reduced Total and Cause-Specific Death Rates in Older Women? The Iowa Women's Health Study." *American Journal of Public Health* 89 (1999): 322–29.

Jansen, M., et al. "Dietary Fiber and Plant Foods in Relation to Colorectal Cancer Mortality: The Seven Countries Study." *International Journal of Cancer* 81 (1999): 174–79.

Kantor, L., et al. "Choose a Variety of Grains Daily, Especially Whole Grains: A Challenge for Consumers." *Journal of Nutrition* 131 (2001): 473S–486S.

Lui, S., et al. "A Prospective Study of Dietary Glycemic Load, Carbohydrate Intake and Risk of Coronary Heart Disease in US Women." *American Journal of Clinical Nutrition* 71 (2000): 1455–461.

Lui, S., et al. "A Prospective Study of Whole-Grain Intake and Risk of Type 2 Diabetes Mellitus in US Women." *American Journal of Public Health* 90 (2000): 1409–15.

Lui, S., et al. "Whole-grain Consumption and Risk of Coronary Heart Disease: Results from the Nurses' Health Study." *American Journal of Clinical Nutrition* 70 (1999): 412–19.

Lui, S., et al. "Whole Grain Consumption and Risk of Ischemic Stroke in Women." *Journal of the American Medical Association* 284 (2000): 1534–40.

Miller, H., et al. "Antioxidant Content of Whole Grain Breakfast Cereals, Fruits and Vegetables." *Journal of the American College of Nutrition* 19 (2000): 312S–319S.

Myer, K., et al. "Carbohydrates, Dietary Fiber, and Incident Type 2 Diabetes in Older Women." *American Journal of Clinical Nutrition* 71 (2000): 921–30.

Slavin, J. "Mechanisms for the Impact of Whole Grain Foods on Cancer Risk." *Journal of the American College of Nutrition* 19 (2000): 300S–307S.

Slavin, J., et al. "Grain Processing and Nutrition." *Critical Reviews in Food Science and Nutrition* 40 (2000): 309–26.

Slavin, J., et al. "Plausible Mechanisms for the Protectiveness of Whole Grains." *American Journal of Clinical Nutrition* 70 (1999): 459S–463S.

Zielinski, H., and Kozlowska, H. "Antioxidant Activity and Total Phenolics in Selected Cereal Grains and Their Different Morphological Fractions." *Journal of Agriculture and Food Chemistry* 48 (2000) 2008–16.

Looking-Good, Low-Fat Milk Products

Chan, J., et al. "Dairy Products, Calcium, and Prostate Cancer Risk in the Physicians' Health Study." *American Journal of Clinical Nutrition* 74 (2001): 549–54.

Davies, M., et al. "Calcium Intake and Body Weight." *The Journal of Clinical Endocrinology and Metabolism* 86 (2000): 4635–38.

Dunne, C., et al. "In Vitro Selection Criteria for Probiotic Bacteria of Human Origin: Correlation with In Vivo Findings." *American Journal of Clinical Nutrition* 73 (2001): 386S–392S.

Garland, D., et al. "Calcium and Vitamin D—Their Potential Roles in Colon and Breast Cancer Prevention." *Annals of New York Academy of Sciences* 889 (1999): 107–19.

Gueguen, L., et al. "The Bioavailability of Dietary Calcium." *Journal of the American College of Nutrition* 19 (2000): 119S–136S.

Heaney, R. "Calcium, Dairy Products and Osteoporosis." *Journal of the American College of Nutrition* 19 (2000): 83S–99S.

Holt, P. "Dairy Foods and Prevention of Colon Cancer: Human Studies." *Journal of the American College of Nutrition* 18 (1999): 379S–391S.

Ilich, J., and Kerstetter, J. "Nutrition in Bone Health Revisited: A Story Beyond Calcium." *Journal of the American College of Nutrition* 19 (2000): 715–37.

Isolauri, E., et al. "Probiotics: Effects on Immunity." *American Journal of Clinical Nutrition* 73 (2001): 444S–450S.

MacDonald, H. "Conjugated Linoleic Acid and Disease Prevention: A Review of Current Knowledge." *Journal of the American College of Nutrition* 19 (2000): 111S–118S.

Maijala, K. "Cow Milk and Human Development and Well-Being." *Livestock Production Science* 65 (2000): 1–18.

McBean, L. "Emerging Dietary Benefits of Dairy Foods." *Nutrition Today* 34 (1999): 47–53.

Miller, G., et al. "Benefits of Dairy Product Consumption on Blood Pressure in Humans: A Summary of the Biomedical Literature." *Journal of the American College of Nutrition* 19 (2000): 147S–164S.

Mobarhan, S. "Calcium and the Colon: Recent Findings." *Nutrition Reviews* 57 (1999): 124–29.

Mombelli, B., and Gismondo, M. "The Use of Probiotics in Medical Practice." *International Journal of Antimicrobial Agents* 16 (2000): 531–36.

National Institute of Health. "Osteoporosis Prevention, Diagnosis and Therapy." *Journal of the American Medical Association* 285 (2001): 785–95.

New, S. "Bone Health: the Role of Micronutrients." *British Medical Bulletin* 55 (1999): 619–33.

Power, M., et al. "The Role of Calcium in Health and Disease." *American Journal of Obstetricians and Gynecologists* 181 (1999): 1560–69.

Raisz, L. "Osteoporosis: Current Approaches and Future Prospects in Diagnosis, Pathogenesis, and Management." *Journal of Bone and Mineral Metabolism* 17 (1999): 79–89.

Stanton, C., et al. "Market Potential for Probiotics." *American Journal of Clinical Nutrition* 73 (2001): 476S–483S.

Vess, T., et al. "Lactose Intolerance." *Journal of the American College of Nutrition* 19 (2000): 165S–175S.

Vieth, R. "Vitamin D Supplementation and Safety." *American Journal of Clinical Nutrition* 69 (1999): 842–56.

Weaver, C., et al. "Choices for Achieving Adequate Dietary Calcium with a Vegetarian Diet." *American Journal for Clinical Nutrition* 70 (1999): 543S–548S.

Weber, P. "The Role of Vitamins in the Prevention of Osteoporosis—A Brief Status Report." *International Journal of Vitamin Nutrition Research* 69 (1999): 194–97.

Weinsier, R., and Krundieck, C. "Dairy Foods and Bone Health: Examination of the Evidence." *American Journal of Clinical Nutrition* 72 (2000): 681–89.

Wosje, K., and Specker, B. "Role of Calcium in Bone Health During Childhood." *Nutrition Reviews* 58 (2000): 253–68.

Sensational Soy and the Whole Darn Bean Family

Adlercreutz, H., et al. "Phytoestrogens and Prostate Disease." *Journal of Nutrition* 130 (2000): 658S–659S.

Anderson, J., et al. "Cardiovascular and Renal Benefits of Dry Bean and Soybean Intake." *American Journal of Clinical Nutrition* 70 (1999): 464S–474S.

Anderson, J., and Hanna, T. "Impact of Nondigestible Carbohydrates on Serum Lipoproteins and Risk for Cardiovascular Disease." *Journal of Nutrition* 129 (1999): 1457S–1466S.

Anthony, M. "Soy and Cardiovascular Disease: Cholesterol Lowering and Beyond." *Journal of Nutrition* 130 (2000): 662S–663S.

Barnes, S., et al. "Isoflavonoids and Chronic Disease: Mechanisms of Action." *Biofactors* 12 (2000): 209–15.

Burke, G., et al. "Soybean Isoflavones as an Alternative to Traditional Hormone Replacement Therapy: Are We There Yet?" *Journal of Nutrition* 130 (2000): 664S–665S.

Cassidy, A., and Faughnan, M. "Phyto-oestrogens Through the Life Cycle." *Proceedings of the Nutrition Society* 59 (2000): 489–96.

Costa, R., and Summa, M. "Soy Protein in the Management of Hyperlipidemia." *The Annals of Pharmacotherapy* 34 (2000): 931–35.

Dunn, A. "Incorporating Soy Protein into a Low-fat, Low-cholesterol Diet." *Cleveland Clinic Journal of Medicine* 67 (2000): 767–71.

Geil, P., and Anderson, J. "Nutrition and Health Implications of Dry Beans: A Review." *Journal of the American College of Nutrition* 13 (1994): 549–58.

Greenwood, S., et al. "The Role of Isoflavones in Menopausal Health: Consensus Opinion of the North American Menopause Society." *The Journal of the North American Menopause Society* 7 (2000): 215–29.

Kurzer, M. "Hormonal Effects of Soy Isoflavones: Studies in Premenopausal and Postmenopausal Women." *Journal of Nutrition* 130 (2000): 660S–661S.

Kushi, L., et al. "Cereals, Legumes, and Chronic Disease Risk Reduction: Evidence from Epidemiologic Studies." *American Journal of Clinical Nutrition* 70 (1999): 451S–458S.

Lamartiniere, C. "Protection Against Breast Cancer with Genistein: A Component of Soy." *American Journal of Clinical Nutrition* 71 (2000): 1705S–1707S.

Messina, M., and Erdman, J. "Third International Symposium on the Role of Soy in Preventing and Treating Chronic Disease." *Journal of Nutrition* 130 (2000): 653S.

Schouw, Y., et al. "Phyto-oestrogens and Cardiovascular Disease Risk." *Nutrition Metabolism and Cardiovascular Disease* 10 (2000): 154–67.

Vincent, A., and Fitzpatrick, L. "Soy Isoflavones: Are They Useful in Menopause?" *Mayo Clinic Proceedings* 75 (2000): 1174–84.

Wakai, K., et al. "Dietary Intake and Sources of Isoflavones Among Japanese." *Nutrition and Cancer* 33 (1999): 139–45.

Wroblewski, L., and Cooke, J. "Phytoestrogens and Cardiovascular Health." *Journal of the American College of Cardiology* 35 (2000): 1403–10.

Fantastic Fish

Bruinsma, K., and Taren, D. "Dieting, Essential Fatty Acid Intake, and Depression." *Nutrition Reviews* 58 (2000): 98–108.

Connor, W. "Importance of Omega-3 Fatty Acids in Health and Disease." *American Journal of Clinical Nutrition* 71 (2000): 171S–175S.

Das, U. "Beneficial Effects of Omega-3 Fatty Acids in Cardiovascular Diseases: But, Why and How?" *Prostaglandins, Leukotrienes and Essential Fatty Acids* 63 (2000): 351–62.

Hibbeln, J., and Salem, N. "Dietary Polyunsaturated Fatty Acids and Depression: When Cholesterol Does not Satisfy." *American Journal of Clinical Nutrition* 62 (1995): 1–9.

Iso, H., et al. "Intake of Fish and Omega-3 Fatty Acids and Risk of Stroke in Women." *Journal of the American Medical Association* 285 (2001): 304–12.

James, M., et al. "Dietary Polyunsaturated Fatty Acids and Inflammatory Mediator Production." *American Journal of Clinical Nutrition* 71 (2000): 343S–348S.

Kremer, J. "Omega-3 Fatty Acid Supplements in Rheumatoid Arthritis." *American Journal of Clinical Nutrition* 71 (2000): 349S–351S.

Marckmann, P., and Gronback, M. "Fish Consumption and Coronary Heart Disease Mortality. A Systematic Review of Prospective Cohort Studies." *European Journal of Clinical Nutrition* 53 (1999): 585–90.

Nestel, P. "Fish Oil and Cardiovascular Disease: Lipids and Arterial Function." *American Journal of Clinical Nutrition* 71 (2000): 228S–231S.

O'Keefe, J., and Harris, W. "From Inuit to Implementation: Omega-3 Fatty Acids Come of Age." *Mayo Clinic Proceedings* 75 (2000): 607–14.

Rose, D., and Connolly, J. "Omega-3 Fatty Acids as Cancer Chemopreventive Agents." *Pharmacology and Therapeutics* 83 (1999): 217–44.

Schacky, C. "Omega-3 Fatty Acids and the Prevention of Coronary Atherosclerosis." *American Journal of Clinical Nutrition* 71 (2000): 224S–227S.

Simopoulos, A. "Human Requirement for Omega-3 Polyunsaturated Fatty Acids." *Poultry Science* 79 (2000): 961–70.

World Health Organization. "Food Safety Issues Associated with Products From Aquaculture." Switzerland: World Health Organization Office of Publications, 1999.

The Meat, Poultry and Egg Story

Hu, F., et al. "A Prospective Study of Egg Consumption and Risk of Cardiovascular Disease in Men and Women." *Journal of the American Medical Association* 281 (1999): 1387–94.

Hu, F., et al. "Dietary Saturated Fats and Their Food Sources in Relation to the Risk of Coronary Heart Disease in Women." *American Journal of Clinical Nutrition* 70 (1999): 1001–08.

Hunningbake, D., et al. "Incorporation of Lean Red Meat into a National Cholesterol Education Program Step I Diet: A Long-Term, Randomized Clinical Trial in Free-Living Persons with Hypercholesterolemia." *Journal of the American College of Nutrition* 19 (2000): 351–60.

Key, T., et al. "Mortality in Vegetarians and Nonvegetarians: Detailed Findings from a Collaborative Analysis of 5 Prospective Studies." *American Journal of Clinical Nutrition* 70 (2000): 516S–524S.

Lewis, N., et al. "Enriched Eggs as a Source of N-3 Polyunsaturated Fatty Acids for Humans." *Poultry Science* 79 (2000): 971–74.

Mann, N. "Dietary Lean Red Meat and Human Evolution." *European Journal of Nutrition* 39 (2000): 71–79.

McNamara, D. "The Impact of Egg Limitations on Coronary Heart Disease Risk: Do the Numbers Add Up?" *Journal of the American College of Nutrition* 19 (2000): 540S–548S.

Nerurkar, P., et al. "Effects of Marinating With Asian Marinades or Western Barbecue Sauce on PhIP and MelQx Formation in Barbecued Beef." *Nutrition and Cancer* 34 (1999): 147–52.

Norat, T., and Riboli, E. "Meat Consumption and Colorectal Cancer: A Review of Epidemiologic Evidence." *Nutrition Reviews* 59 (2001): 37–47.

Platz, E., et al. "Proportion of Colon Cancer Risk that Might Be Preventable in a Cohort of Middle-Aged US Men." *Cancer Causes and Control* 11 (2000): 579–88.

Tavani, A. "Red Meat Intake and Cancer Risk: A Study in Italy." *International Journal of Cancer* 86 (2000): 425–28.

Weggemans, R. "Dietary Cholesterol from Eggs Increases the Ratio of Total Cholesterol to High-Density Lipoprotein Cholesterol in Humans: A Meta-Analysis." *American Journal of Clinical Nutrition* 73 (2001): 885–991.

Yoon, H., et al. "Systematic Review of Epidemiological Studies on Meat, Dairy Products and Egg Consumption and Risk of Colorectal Adenomas." *European Journal of Cancer Prevention* 9 (2000): 151–64.

Go Nuts!

Hu, F., et al. "Frequent Nut Consumption and Risk of Coronary Heart Disease in Women: Prospective Cohort Study." *British Medical Journal* 317 (1998): 1341–45.

Hu, F., and Stampfer, M. "Nut Consumption and Risk of Coronary Heart Disease: A Review of Epidemiologic Evidence." *Current Atherosclerosis Reports* 1 (1999): 205–10.

Kris-Etherton, P., et al. "High-Monounsaturated Fatty Acid Diets Lower Both Plasma Cholesterol and Triacylglycerol Concentrations." *American Journal of Clinical Nutrition* 70 (1999): 1009–15.

Kris-Etherton, P., et al. "Nuts and Their Bioactive Constituents: Effects on Serum Lipids and Other Factors That Affect Disease Risk." *American Journal of Clinical Nutrition* 70 (1999): 504S–511S.

Sabate, J. "Nut Consumption, Vegetarian Diets, Ischemic Heart Disease Risk, and All-cause Mortality: Evidence from Epidemiologic Studies." *American Journal of Clinical Nutrition* 70 (1999): 500S–503S.

Fabulous Flax

Cunnane, S., et al. "High Alpha-linolenic Acid Flaxseed: Some Nutritional Properties in Humans." *British Journal of Nutrition* 69 (1993): 443–53.

Cunnane, S., et al. "Nutritional Attributes of Traditional Flaxseed in Healthy Young Adults." *American Journal of Clinical Nutrition* 61 (1995): 62–68.

Demark-Wahnefried, W., et al. "Pilot Study of Dietary Fat Restriction and Flaxseed Supplementation in Men with Prostate Cancer Before Surgery: Exploring the Effect on Hormonal Levels, Prostate-Specific Antigen and Histopathologic Features." *Urology* 58 (2001): 47–52.

Haggans, C., et al. "Effect of Flaxseed Consumption on Urinary Estrogen Metabolites in Postmenopausal Women." *Nutrition and Cancer* 33 (1999): 188–95.

Hutchins, A., et al. "Flaxseed Influences Urinary Lignan Excretion in a Dose-Dependent Manner in Postmenopausal Women." *Cancer Epidemiology Biomarkers Prevention* 10 (2000): 1113–18.

Jenkins, D., et al. "Health Aspects of Partially Defatted Flaxseed, Including Effects on Serum Lipids, Oxidative Measures, and Ex Vivo Androgen and Progestin Activity: A Controlled Crossover Trial." *American Journal of Clinical Nutrition* 69 (1999): 395–402.

Nesbitt, P., and Thompson, L. "Lignans in Homemade and Commercial Products Containing Flaxseed." *Nutrition and Cancer* 29 (1997): 222–27.

Time for Tea

Ahmad, N., and Mukhtar, H. "Green Tea Polyphenols and Cancer: Biologic mechanisms and Practical Implications." *Nutrition Reviews* 57 (1999): 78–82.

Ahmad, N., and Mukhtar, H. "Tea Polyphenols: Prevention of Cancer and Optimizing Health." *American Journal of Clinical Nutrition* 71 (2000): 1698S–1702S.

Dulloo, A., et al. "Efficacy of a Green Tea Extract Rich in Catechin Polyphenols and Caffeine in Increasing 24 hour Energy Expenditure and Fat Oxidation in Humans." *American Journal of Clinical Nutrition* 70 (1999): 1040–45.

Hodgson, J., et al. "Acute Effects of Ingestion of Black and Green Tea on Lipoprotein Oxidation." *American Journal of Clinical Nutrition* 71 (2000): 1103–07.

Hollman, P., et al. "Tea Flavonols in Cardiovascular Disease and Cancer Epidemiology." *Experimental Biology and Medicine* 220 (1999): 198–202.

Phipps, R. "The Second International Scientific Symposium on Tea & Human Health." *Nutrition* 15 (1999): 968–71.

Pip, E. "Survey of Bottled Drinking Water Available in Manitoba, Canada." *Environmental Health Perspectives* 108 (2000): 863–66.

Riemersma, R., et al. "Tea Flavonoids and Cardiovascular Health." *QJM: Monthly Journal of the Association of Physicians* 94 (2001): 277–82.

Trevisanato, S., and Young-In, K. "Tea and Health." *Nutrition Reviews* 58 (2000): 1–10.

Weisburger, J. "Tea and Health: The Underlying Mechanisms." *Experimental Biology and Medicine* 220 (1999): 271–75.

Yang, C., and Landau, J. "Effects of Tea Consumption on Nutrition and Health." *Journal of Nutrition* 130 (2000): 2409–12.

What About Wine?

Ajani, U., et al. "Alcohol Consumption and Risk of Coronary Heart Disease by Diabetes Status." *Circulation* 102 (2000): 500–05.

Berger, K., et al. "Light-to-Moderate Alcohol Consumption and the Risk of Stroke Among U.S. Male Physicians." *The New England Journal of Medicine* 341 (1999): 1557–64.

Das, D., et al. "Cardioprotection of Red Wine: Role of Polyphenolic Antioxidants." *Drugs, Experimenal and Clinical Research* 2/3 (1999): 115–20.

Doll, R. "One for the Heart." *British Medical Journal* 315 (1997): 1664–68.

Flesch, M., et al. "Alcohol and the Risk of Myocardial Infarction." *Basic Research in Cardiology* 96 (2001): 128–35.

Fuchs, C., et al. "Alcohol Consumption and Mortality Among Women." *The New England Journal of Medicine* 332 (1995): 1245–50.

Gaziano, J., et al. "Light-to-Moderate Alcohol Consumption and Mortality in the Physicians' Health Study Enrollment Cohort." *Journal of the American College of Cardiology* 35 (2000): 531–38.

German, J., and Walzem, R. "The Health Benefits of Wine." *Annual Reviews in Nutrition* 20 (2000): 561–93.

Goldberg, D., et al. "Moderate Alcohol Consumption: The Gentle Face of Janus." *Clinical Biochemistry* 32 (1999): 505–18.

Grenbaek, M., et al. "Type of Alcohol Consumed and Mortality from All Causes, Coronary Heart Disease and Cancer." *Annals of Internal Medicine* 133 (2000): 411–19.

Puddey, I., and Croft, K. "Alcohol, Stroke and Coronary Heart Disease." *Neuroepidemiology* 18 (1999): 292–302.

Rehm, J., and Bondy, S. "Alcohol and All-Cause Mortality: An Overview." *Novartis Foundation Symposium* (1998): 223–36.

Rimm, E., et al. "Moderate Alcohol Intake and Lower Risk of Coronary Heart Disease: Meta-Analysis of Effects on Lipids and Haemostatic Factors." *British Medical Journal* 319 (1999): 1523–28.

Ruf, J. "Wine and Polyphenols Related to Platelet Aggregation and Atherothrombosis." *Drugs, Experimental and Clinical Research* 2/3 (1999): 125–31.

Thun, M., et al. "Alcohol Consumption and Mortality Among Middle-Aged and Elderly U.S. Adults." *The New England Journal of Medicine* 337 (1997): 1705–14.

Tsugane, S., et al. "Alcohol Consumption and All-Cause Mortality among Middle-aged Japanese Men: Seven-year Follow-up of the JPHC Study Cohort." *American Journal of Epidemiology* 150 (1999): 1201–07.

Sacco, R., et al. "The Protective Effect of Moderate Alcohol Consumption on Ischemic Stroke." *Journal of the American Medical Association* 281 (1999): 53–60.

Vinson, J., et al. "Red Wine, Dealcoholized Red Wine, and Especially Grape Juice, Inhibit Atherosclerosis in a Hamster Model." *Atherosclerosis* 156 (2000): 67–72.

The Nutritional Supplement Debate

Eichholzer, M. et al. "The Role of Folate, Antioxidant Vitamins and Other Constituents in Fruit and Vegetables in the Prevention of Cardiovascular Disease: The Epidemiological Evidence." *International Journal of Vitamin Nutrition Research* 71 (2001): 5–17.

Giovannucci, E. et al. "Multivitamin Use, Folate, and Colon Cancer in Women in the Nurses' Health Study." *Annals of Internal Medicine* 129 (1998): 517–24.

Jialal, I., et al. "Is There a Vitamin E Paradox?" *British Medical Journal* 12 (2001): 49–53.

Maxwell, S. "Coronary Artery Disease—Free Radical Damage, Antioxidant Protection and the Role of Homocysteine." *Basic Research In Cardiology* 95 (2000): 65S–71S.

McDermott, J. "Antioxidant Nutrients: Current Dietary Recommendations and Research Update." *Journal of the American Pharmaceutical Association* 40 (2000): 785–99.

Rimm, E., et al. "Folate and Vitamin B6 from Diet and Supplements in Relation to Coronary Heart Disease Among Women." *Journal of the American Medical Association* 5 (1998): 359–64.

Tran, T. "Antioxidant Supplements to Prevent Heart Disease." *Postgraduate Medicine* 109 (2001): 109–14.

Active Living for a Lifetime

AHA Science Advisory. "Resistance Exercise in Individuals with and without Cardiovascular Disease." *Circulation* 101 (2000): 828.

McInnis, K. "Exercise and Obesity." *Coronary Artery Disease* 11 (2000): 111–16.

Rippe, J. and Hess, S. "The Role of Physical Activity in the Prevention and Management of Obesity." *Journal of the American Dietetic Association* 98 (1998): S31–S38.

NUTRITION INFORMATION INDEX

RECIPE INDEX

ABOUT THE AUTHORS

liz pearson

Liz Pearson isn't afraid to admit that she loves chocolate as much as the next person. Her ability to communicate timely, relevant nutrition research, while emphasizing the need for fun food in moderation is what makes her approach to healthy eating so sane and sensible. Liz's first book, *When in Doubt, Eat Broccoli! (But Leave Some Room for Chocolate)* received outstanding reviews from consumers and health professionals alike.

Born and raised in Toronto, Liz is a Registered Dietitian. She received her Bachelor of Applied Arts Degree in Nutrition from Ryerson Polytechnic University and completed her dietetic internship at the Toronto General Hospital. Now one of Canada's most high profile nutrition experts, Liz is an in-demand speaker for both health professionals and consumers.

Liz runs The Pearson Institute of Nutrition, which converts pertinent nutrition research into a format consumers can understand and use in their busy lives. She is also the spokes-person for the 5-to-10-a-day fruit and vegetable campaign sponsored by The Heart and Stroke Foundation of Canada and the Canadian Cancer Society, and the nutrition expert for *Chatelaine* magazine.

mairlyn smith

A multi-talented home economist, teacher and actor, Mairlyn Smith loves to add a dash of comedy to her cooking. Born in Vancouver, Mairlyn graduated in 1976 with a degree in Home Economics from the University of British Columbia. She then returned to UBC and completed her Teaching Certificate, going on to teach Home Economics and head the Department of Fine Arts at Balmoral Junior High.

Unable to shake the acting bug, Mairlyn enrolled at the American Academy of Dramatic Arts in California. Then, she moved to Toronto to find work. Mairlyn has amassed an impressive resume of credits: she is the author of *Lick the Spoon!*, an alumnis of Second City, and a teacher at Loblaw's cooking school in Ontario. Her versatility in acting and cooking with a comedic flair also landed her the job as a host of *Harrowsmith Country Life* and a subsequent Gemini Nomination.

Mairlyn is a film and television performer and does extensive voice-over work for both radio and TV. She is currently working on her next book, *You Are What You Eat and I Ought to Know!*